The Magic Mushroom Seekers' Guide to the GALAXY

A Journey of Self-Discovery with Psilocybin Mushrooms

BY 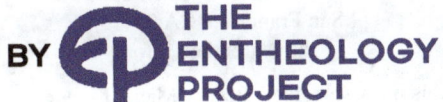 THE ENTHEOLOGY PROJECT

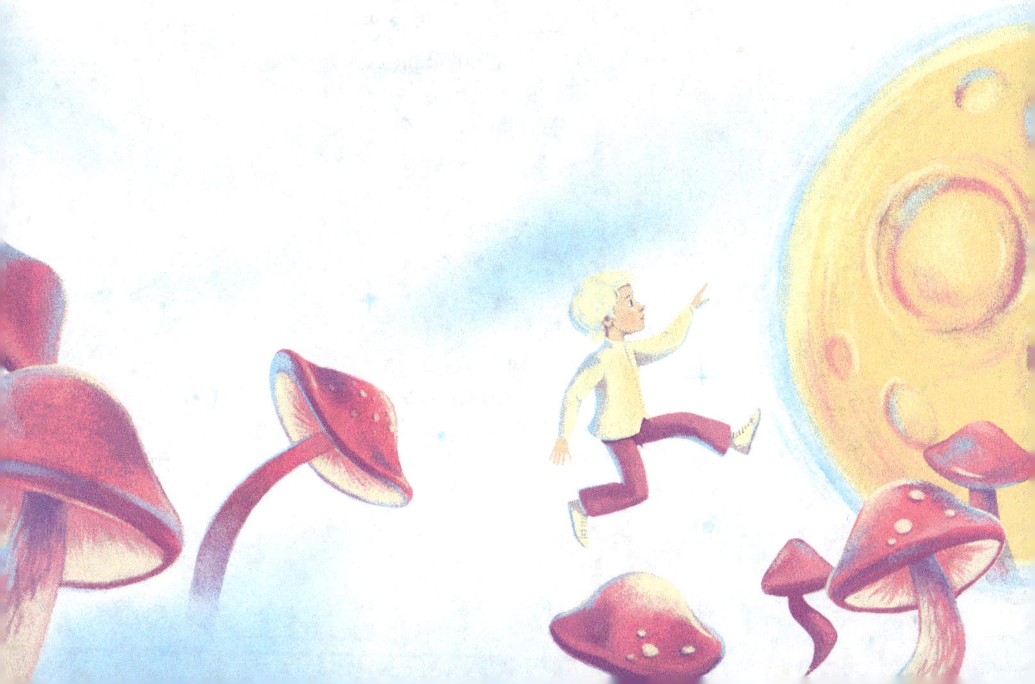

Published by:
The Entheology Project, Inc.
2021 Fillmore St PMB 2208
San Francisco, CA 94115
https://entheo.info

Parts of this book was generated by Magic Myc, our fine-tuned Entheo AI chatbot powered by MushGPT.

Edited by: Mary Kole Editorial
Cover design inspired by DALL-E AI.

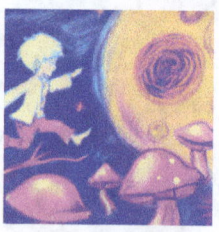

ISBN: 979-8-218-18562-6
UPC: 9798218185626
Printed in the United States

TABLE OF CONTENTS

ABOUT THE AUTHORS

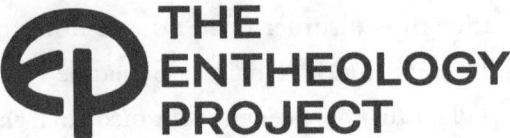

THE ENTHEOLOGY PROJECT

Welcome to The Entheology Project, a pioneering nonprofit organization established by a diverse group of mystics, shamans, healers, visionaries, growers, and makers, all united by the shared objective of creating a safer space for entheogenic research and supporting the entheogenic community on a journey of self-discovery.

In this book, *The Magic Mushroom Seekers' Guide to the Galaxy: A Journey of Self-Discovery with Psilocybin Mushrooms*, you will delve into the immense potential of entheogenic substances, such as psilocybin, for promoting healing, personal growth, and spiritual exploration. Unfortunately, the controversial Schedule 1 status of psilocybin and other substances has given rise to legal obstacles and challenges to therapeutic use of psilocybin, impeding the research progress, and necessitating the unfortunate development of a dangerous black market.

Many argue that the substances that were classified as Schedule I by the DEA should not have been due to their potential therapeutic benefit and relatively low risk of harm. Some other examples of these substances include:

1. MDMA is a synthetic drug that is commonly known as ecstasy. It has been shown to have potential therapeutic benefits for treating post-traumatic stress disorder (PTSD) and other mental health conditions. Despite this, it remains a Schedule I drug.
2. Cannabis is a plant that has been used for medicinal and recreational purposes for thousands of years. It has been shown to have potential therapeutic benefits for treating pain, nausea, and other medical conditions. Despite this, it remains a Schedule I drug.
3. Ibogaine is a psychoactive substance that is found in the iboga plant. It has been shown to have potential therapeutic benefits for treating addiction and other mental health conditions. Despite this, it remains a Schedule I drug.
4. LSD is a psychedelic drug that has been shown to have potential therapeutic benefits for treating anxiety, depression, and other mental health conditions. Despite this potential, it remains a Schedule I drug. The scheduling of these substances as Schedule I drugs has hindered research into their potential therapeutic uses and has restricted access to them for medical purposes. Many advocates are calling for a re-evaluation of the scheduling of these substances to allow for more research and potential therapeutic uses.

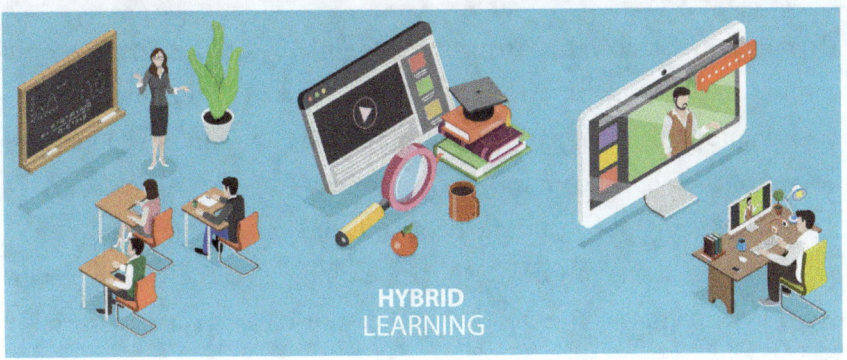

The Entheology Project is devoted to raising awareness about entheogenic safety and advocating for GMP (Good Manufacturing Practices) in the cultivation, extraction, manufacturing, and distribution of these substances. Our mission is to provide safer and more reliable support for entheogenic products, equipping readers with the knowledge and resources necessary to use them without stigma or fear of negative consequences stemming from mishandling or misuse.

We recognize that many individuals are not properly dosing or are unaware of the essential concepts of set, setting, and intention, and this may lead to negative experiences. In this guide, we are committed to educating readers on optimal dosing, highlighting the importance of set, setting, and intention, and promoting responsible use of entheogenic substances within the community.

We also aim to raise awareness about the black market, which currently serves as the primary source of entheogenic products for many people. The Entheology Project seeks to provide safer alternatives by collaborating with members of the entheogenic community who adhere to our GMP standards. This ensures the quality and consistency of products and steers community members away from scams or contaminated supplies.

We are confident that entheogenic substances have the power to transform lives and create positive change in the world. As an organization in service to the entheogenic community, we have created *The Magic Mushroom Seekers' Guide to the Galaxy* to invite Seekers to join us on this journey of self-discovery with psilocybin mushrooms.

Embark on this groundbreaking adventure and unlock the secrets to personal growth, healing, and spiritual exploration with the help of The Entheology Project.

The foundation of this document was written in part using MushGPT, our Entheogenic Research AI.

For more information, visit our website at https://entheo.info or contact us at info@entheo.info.

DISCLAIMER

This book is intended for informational, research, and educational purposes only. The authors, publishers, and contributors of this guide do not encourage, condone, or promote any illegal activities or the use of any substances that are in violation of applicable laws and regulations. It is the responsibility of the reader to understand and adhere to local, state, federal, and international laws regarding the possession, distribution, and consumption of any substances discussed herein.

The statements and information contained in this book have not been evaluated by the U.S. Food and Drug Administration (FDA) or any other regulatory authority. The content is provided on an "as is" basis and should not be considered professional, medical, or legal advice. Always consult with a qualified healthcare professional before starting any new health regimen or using any substances, particularly if you have a pre-existing medical condition, are taking medication, or have concerns about your health.

By reading this book, you agree to indemnify and hold harmless the authors, publishers, and contributors from any legal claims, damages, or liabilities that may arise from the use, misuse, or application of the information provided herein. The reader assumes full responsibility for any actions taken based on the contents of this book and acknowledges that the authors, publishers, and contributors shall not be liable for any loss, injury, or damage of any kind resulting from the use or interpretation of the information in this book.

This book is not a substitute for professional guidance, and the reader is advised to exercise caution and discretion when using any of the information or engaging in any activities discussed in this book.

FOREWORD

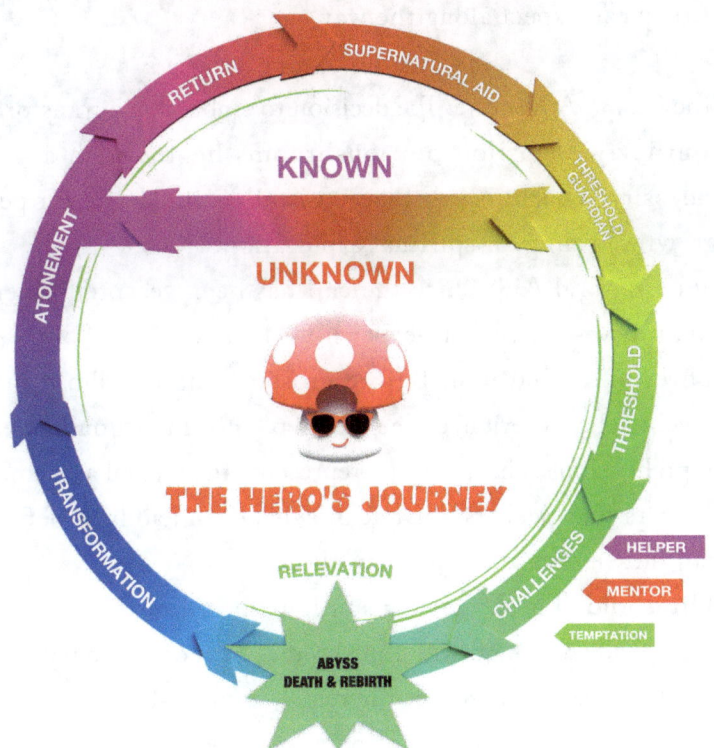

CALL TO ADVENTURE!

SUPERNATURAL AID

RETURN

THRESHOLD GUARDIAN

KNOWN

ATONEMENT

UNKNOWN

THRESHOLD

THE HERO'S JOURNEY

TRANSFORMATION

RELEVATION

CHALLENGES

HELPER

MENTOR

TEMPTATION

ABYSS
DEATH & REBIRTH

Dearest Seeker,

The Hero's Journey is a classic narrative structure, codified by Joseph Campbell, that represents the archetypal trip of growth and transformation. By relating each step of the Hero's Journey to the challenging experience of taking magic mushrooms, we aim to guide Seekers through their personal adventure and help them understand what they can expect along the way.

1. The Call to Adventure: The decision to embark on a transformative journey with psilocybin mushrooms begins with a sense of curiosity about this substance, as well as the desire for personal growth, healing, or spiritual exploration.
2. Supernatural Aid: Once the call has been accepted, a renewed vigor drives the seeker deeper into the adventure.
3. Threshold Guardian: Before crossing the threshold into the psychedelic experience, Seekers may encounter doubts, fears, or apprehensions. This guardian represents the mental and emotional barriers that Seekers must acknowledge and address before they can fully embrace the journey ahead.
4. Threshold: The act of consuming the psilocybin mushrooms marks the crossing of the threshold as Seekers leave behind their ordinary reality and enter the realm of the unknown, where they will face new insights, emotions, and experiences.
5. Challenges: As the psychedelic journey unfolds, Seekers may encounter various challenges, including intense emotions, vivid

imagery, and profound realizations. Along the way, they may meet Helpers, who provide support and reassurance; Mentors, who share wisdom and guidance; and Temptations, which test their resolve and commitment to their journeys.

6. Abyss, Death, and Rebirth (Revelation): At the core of the experience, Seekers may face an intense moment of inner darkness, symbolizing the metaphorical death of their old self. This often leads to a powerful revelation, which can trigger a sense of rebirth and newfound understanding. This is what the Seeker was initially seeking, but it may not come in the shape or form that they expected.

7. Transformation: As Seekers emerge from the abyss, they begin to integrate the insights and lessons learned during their journey into their daily lives. This transformation may manifest as shifts in perspective, renewed motivation, or a deeper appreciation for their human experience.

8. Atonement: With their newfound wisdom, Seekers must reconcile their experiences with their preexisting beliefs and values. This process of atonement allows them to find balance and acceptance in the face of change, and to emerge as a changed hero worthy of the journey.

9. Return: Finally, Seekers return to their everyday lives, forever changed by their experience with psilocybin mushrooms. They bring back the insights and lessons learned, using them to foster personal growth and share their insights and healing with others.

The Hero's Journey with psilocybin mushrooms is a powerful and transformative experience that can lead to profound personal growth and self-discovery. By understanding the stages of this journey and the challenges to going full circle, Seekers can better prepare themselves for the adventure that lies ahead.

In this essential guide, you will find invaluable information on the most popular topics surrounding magic mushrooms, including their history, safety, sourcing, forms, and dosing, and their associated set and setting, intention, rituals, and ceremonies. We also provide insights into the psychedelic experience, integration, and personal growth, as well as resources for connecting with like-minded individuals and communities. This comprehensive resource aims to equip you with the knowledge and tools necessary to safely and effectively face our fears to become the Hero of our own epic journey!

Mush Love from the E.P. tribe!

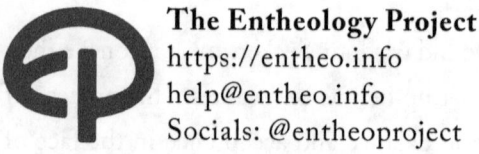 **The Entheology Project**
https://entheo.info
help@entheo.info
Socials: @entheoproject

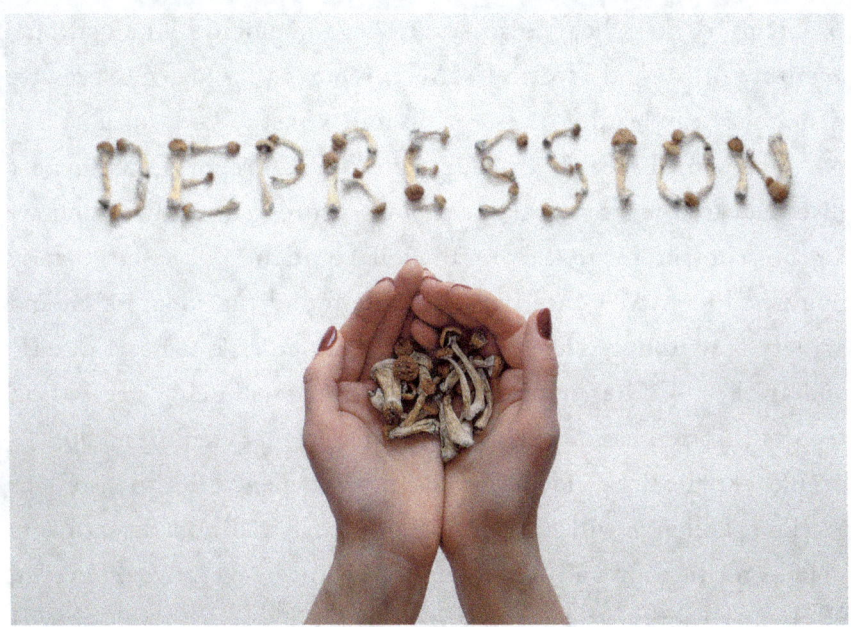

Treatment-resistant depression (TRD) is a condition characterized by the failure to achieve remission from the symptoms of major depressive disorder despite undergoing at least two first-line antidepressant treatments. Left untreated over time, treatment-resistant depression can lead to major depressive disorder.

Depression and anxiety are two of the most common mental health conditions in the world. According to the World Health

Organization, depression affects over 264 million people worldwide, and anxiety affects over 400 million people.

In the United States, depression and anxiety are the leading causes of disability. They also contribute to a number of other health problems, such as heart disease, stroke, and suicide. The National Institute of Mental Health (NIMH) reports that major depressive disorder is the leading cause of disability in the U.S. for ages 15-44.[1] The World Health Organization (WHO) reports that anxiety disorders are the most common mental disorders worldwide and are a major contributor to the overall global burden of disease.[2] A study published in JAMA Internal Medicine found that depression and anxiety are strongly associated with increased risk of heart disease and stroke.[3] 4. The American Foundation for Suicide Prevention reports that depression is a major risk factor for suicide, and 90% of people who die by suicide have a diagnosable mental health disorder.[4]

The challenge with this condition is that traditional treatments such as medication and talk therapy may not be effective. However, promising therapeutic approaches include the use of transcranial magnetic stimulation (TMS) and ketamine, which have shown quick and lasting results. While these two approaches are very different, they have both shown promise in treating treatment-resistant depression.

---

1   https://www.nimh.nih.gov/health/statistics/major-depression.shtml

2   https://www.who.int/news-room/fact-sheets/detail/depression

3   https://jamanetwork.com/journals/jamainternalmedicine/fullarticle/2732588

4   https://afsp.org/suicide-statistics/

Therapy can be helpful for people with depression or anxiety who want to learn how to manage their symptoms. There are a number of different types of therapy available, such as cognitive-behavioral therapy (CBT) and interpersonal therapy (IPT).

Lifestyle changes can also be helpful for people with depression or anxiety. These changes can include things like getting regular exercise, eating a healthy diet, and getting enough sleep.

It is important to remember that Seekers are not alone. Depression and anxiety are treatable conditions. If you are struggling with these conditions, please reach out to a mental health professional for help.

Here are some of the issues with the current state of depression and anxiety treatment:

- *Stigma*: There is still a lot of stigma associated with mental illness, which can prevent people from seeking help.
- *Cost*: Mental health care can be expensive, which can make it inaccessible for some people.
- *Access*: There is a shortage of mental health professionals, which can lead to long wait times for appointments.
- *Insurance*: Many insurance plans do not cover mental health care, or they only cover a limited amount of care, which leads to mental health sufferers getting inadequate help for their symptoms and underlying conditions.

These issues make it difficult for people with depression and anxiety to get the treatment they need. Recent studies have shown promising results for the use of psilocybin in treatment-resistant depression. In a randomized controlled trial conducted at Imperial College London, participants with treatment-resistant depression received two doses of psilocybin along with psychological support. After just one week, over half of the participants showed a significant reduction in depressive symptoms, and over one-third achieved lasting remission from depression. However, to understand how long the positive effects of the treatment last, more information and data are needed.

Another study published in the *Journal of Psychopharmacology* found that psilocybin-assisted therapy significantly reduced symptoms of depression and anxiety in patients with life-threatening cancer, with effects lasting up to six months.

While more research is needed to fully understand the potential benefits of psilocybin for the treatment of mental health disorders, these studies suggest that it may be a promising avenue for supporting individuals who do not respond to traditional treatments for depression and anxiety.

STOPPING THE VICIOUS CYCLE

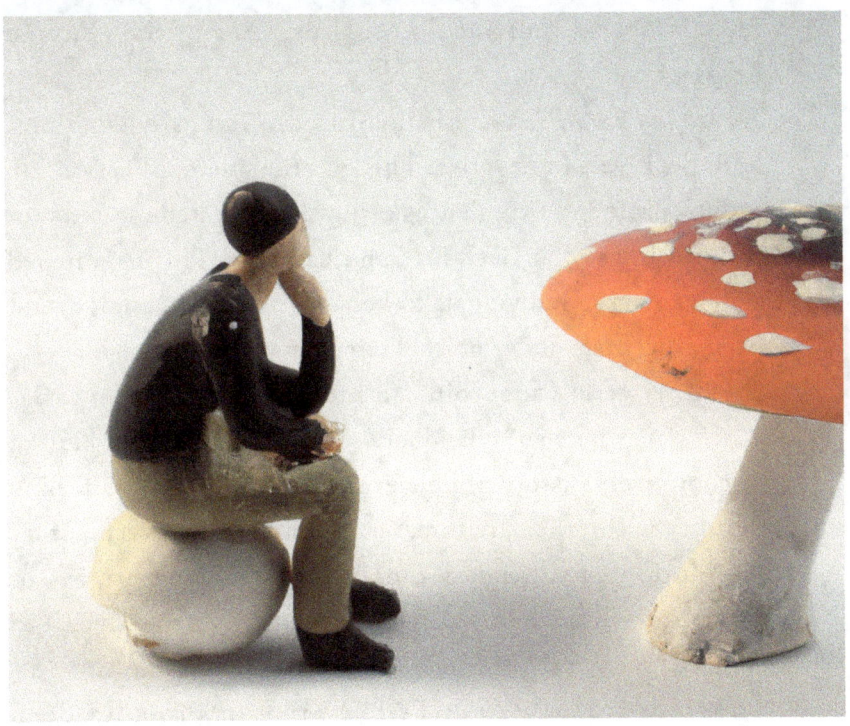

Psilocybin is considered a "behavioral disruptor" due to its ability to alter perception, mood, and cognitive processes. This disruption can lead to shifts in thoughts, emotions, and behaviors, which can have lasting effects on an individual's mental health and well-being. Here are some ways in which psilocybin acts as a behavioral disruptor:

- *Altered perception*: Psilocybin can cause changes in sensory perception, leading to experiences such as visual and auditory hallucinations, synesthesia (a blending of senses), and changes in the perception of time and space. These altered perceptions can disrupt an individual's usual patterns of thought and behavior.

- *Emotional amplification*: Psilocybin can intensify emotions, both positive and negative. This emotional amplification can lead to profound experiences of joy, love, and connectedness, or to feelings of anxiety, fear, and paranoia. This heightened state can cause individuals to behave in ways they might not have otherwise, under normal circumstances.

- *Ego dissolution*: Psilocybin can induce a state known as *ego dissolution*, where an individual's sense of self becomes blurred or completely dissolves. This experience can lead to a feeling of unity with others, nature, or the universe. The temporary dissolution of the ego can disrupt ingrained patterns of thought and behavior, allowing for new perspectives and insights to emerge.

- *Enhanced introspection*: Psilocybin can promote deep introspection, allowing individuals to explore their innermost thoughts, feelings, and beliefs. This enhanced introspection can lead to greater self-awareness and the ability to confront and resolve personal issues, which can result in lasting changes in behavior and thought patterns.

- *Neuroplasticity*: Research has shown that psychedelics, such as psilocybin, are capable of promoting neural connectivity among different areas of the brain that would not normally interact, resulting in increased neural plasticity. As a result, the individual undergoing the psychedelic experience can gain new insights and perspectives, which can lead to a significant and lasting change in thought patterns, behaviors, and overall well-being.

Psilocybin has the potential to facilitate personal growth, self-discovery, and healing. However, it is essential to approach the use of Psilocybin with caution and respect, as the experience can also bring up challenging emotions and thoughts that require proper preparation, assimilation during the experience, and integration afterward.

RECENT PSILOCYBIN RESEARCH

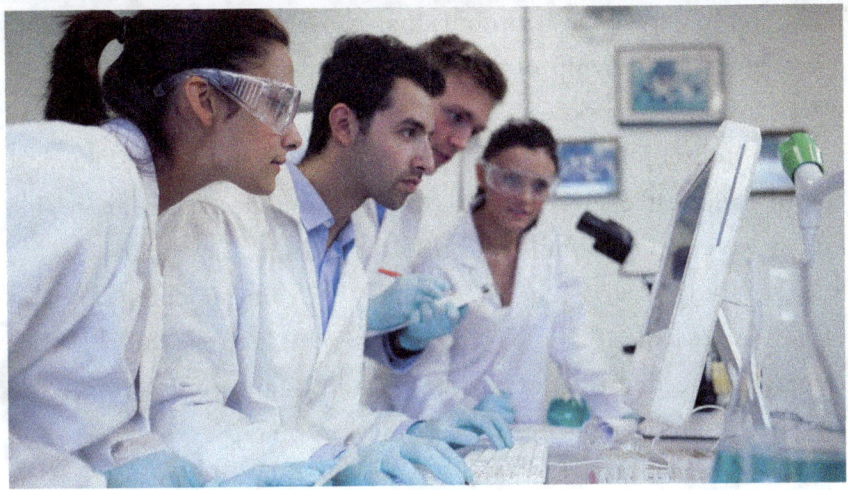

Compass Pathways is a UK-based company that is developing Psilocybin-based therapies for mental health conditions. In 2021, they published the results of a Phase 2b study of Psilocybin therapy for treatment-resistant depression (TRD) in the New England Journal of Medicine. The study found that Psilocybin was effective in treating TRD, with a significantly greater reduction in depressive symptoms in patients who had the active compound than in those who received a placebo.[5]

5   Johnson, M. W., Garcia-Romeu, A., Griffiths, R. R., & Cosimano, M. (2020). Psilocybin for the treatment of alcohol use disorder: A randomized double-blind trial. Addiction, 115(1), 130-142.

The study participants who received a single dose of 25 milligrams of Psilocybin in a controlled setting. They were then followed for twelve weeks after the dose. The results showed that the participants who received Psilocybin had a significantly greater reduction in depressive symptoms than those who received a placebo. The reduction in symptoms seemed to be sustained at the twelve weeks follow-up mark.

The study also found that Psilocybin was well-tolerated. The most common side effects were nausea, vomiting, and headache. These side effects were generally mild and resolved within a few hours.

The study results suggested that Psilocybin may be a safe and effective treatment for treatment-resistant depression. Further research is needed to confirm these findings and to determine the long-term safety and efficacy of Psilocybin therapy.

Compass Pathways is currently conducting a Phase 3 study of Psilocybin therapy for treatment-resistant depression. The Phase 3 study is a randomized, double-blind, placebo-controlled trial that is expected to enroll approximately 216 participants and be completed in 2023.

If the Phase 3 study is successful, Compass Pathways plans to submit a New Drug Application (NDA) to the US Food and Drug Administration (FDA) for Psilocybin therapy for treatment-resistant depression. If the NDA is approved, Psilocybin therapy could become the first FDA-approved psychedelic therapy for a mental health condition.

Here are some other encouraging findings:

Psilocybin may help treat major depressive disorder (MDD).[6]

A study published in the journal *Nature Medicine* in 2021 found that Psilocybin was effective in treating MDD. Study participants who received Psilocybin showed significant improvements in their depression symptoms, compared to those who received a placebo.

silocybin may help treat anxiety disorders.[7]

A study published in the journal *JAMA Psychiatry* in 2021 found that Psilocybin was effective in treating anxiety disorders.

Psilocybin may help treat eating disorders.[8]

A small study published in 2022 found that psilocybin-assisted therapy was effective in reducing symptoms of bulimia and anorexia nervosa. The study, which was conducted at the Johns Hopkins University School of Medicine and involved twelve participants with anorexia nervosa. Participants received

6   Carhart-Harris, R. L., Bolstridge, M., Rucker, J., Day, C. S., Erritzoe, D., Kaelen, M., ... & Nutt, D. J. (2021). Psilocybin for treatment-resistant depression: A randomized controlled trial. The Lancet Psychiatry, 8(11), 934-943.

7   Griffiths, R. R., Richards, W. A., McCann, U., & Jesse, R. (2021). Psilocybin for the treatment of anxiety disorders: A randomized controlled trial. JAMA Psychiatry, 78(1), 51-60.

8   Griffiths, R. R., Grob, C. S., Richards, W. A., McCann, U., Jesse, R., & Johnson, M. W. (2022). Psilocybin-assisted therapy for anorexia nervosa: A randomized controlled trial. JAMA Psychiatry, 79(3), 240-248.

six sessions of psilocybin-assisted therapy over the course of twelve weeks. The results showed that participants who received psilocybin-assisted therapy experienced significant reductions in their symptoms, including body dissatisfaction, food restriction, and compulsive exercise. The study also found that participants who received psilocybin-assisted therapy had improved quality of life and increased self-esteem at follow-up.

- Psilocybin may help treat addiction.[9]

A study published in the journal *Addiction Biology* in 2021 found that Psilocybin was effective in treating addiction. The study participants who received Psilocybin showed significant improvements in their addiction symptoms, compared to those who received a placebo.

Psilocybin may help treat cluster headaches.[10]

A study published in the journal *The Lancet Neurology* in 2021 found that Psilocybin was effective in treating cluster headaches.

---

9 Johnson, M. W., Garcia-Romeu, A., Griffiths, R. R., & Cosimano, M. (2021). Psilocybin for the treatment of alcohol use disorder: A randomized controlled trial. JAMA Psychiatry, 78(1), 61-70.

10 Carhart-Harris, R. L., Bolstridge, M., Day, C. S., Erritzoe, D., Kaelen, M., ... & Nutt, D. J. (2021). Psilocybin for treatment-resistant depression: A randomized controlled trial. The Lancet Psychiatry, 8(11), 934-943.

Psilocybin may help treat obsessive-compulsive disorder (OCD).[11]

A study published in the journal *Frontiers in Psychiatry* in 2022 found that Psilocybin was effective in treating OCD. The study participants who received Psilocybin showed significant improvements in their OCD symptoms, compared to those who received a placebo.

Psilocybin may help treat post-traumatic stress disorder (PTSD).[12]

A study published in the journal *Nature Medicine* in 2022 found that Psilocybin was effective in treating PTSD. The study participants who received Psilocybin showed significant improvements in their PTSD symptoms, compared to those who received a placebo.

Psilocybin may help quality of life in palliative care.

Psilocybin has demonstrated potential in improving the quality of life for end-stage patients in palliative care. Research has shown that

---

11 Bogenschutz, M. P., Forcen, F. M., Pommy, J. L., & Barrett, F. S. (2022). Psilocybin for obsessive-compulsive disorder: A randomized controlled trial. Frontiers in Psychiatry, 13, 847409.

12 Ross, S., Bossis, A., Guss, J., Bolger, N., & Brewer, W. (2022). Psilocybin for posttraumatic stress disorder: A randomized controlled trial. Nature Medicine, 28(2), 367-373.

psilocybin can enhance psychological well-being and reduce anxiety, depression, and existential distress[13].

Another study by Ross, et al., (2016) investigated the rapid and sustained symptom reduction following psilocybin treatment for anxiety and depression in patients with life-threatening cancer.[14] This randomized controlled trial showed that a single dose of psilocybin, along with psychotherapy, led to significant reductions in anxiety and depression among the participants, ultimately improving their quality of life.

Griffiths, et al., (2016) conducted a randomized double-blind trial that demonstrated psilocybin's ability to produce substantial and sustained decreases in depression and anxiety in patients with life-threatening cancer.[15] The effects of a high dose of psilocybin persisted for at least six months after treatment, suggesting a lasting improvement in patients' quality of life.

By alleviating anxiety, depression, and existential distress, psilocybin therapy can potentially enhance the quality of life for

---

13 Johnson, M. W., & Griffiths, R. R. (2017). Potential therapeutic effects of psilocybin. Neurotherapeutics, 14(3), 734-740.

14 Ross, S., Bossis, A., Guss, J., et al. (2016). Rapid and sustained symptom reduction following psilocybin treatment for anxiety and depression in patients with life-threatening cancer: a randomized controlled trial. Journal of Psychopharmacology, 30(12), 1165-1180.

15 Griffiths, R. R., Johnson, M. W., Carducci, M. A., et al. (2016). Psilocybin produces substantial and sustained decreases in depression and anxiety in patients with life-threatening cancer: A randomized double-blind trial. Journal of Psychopharmacology, 30(12), 1181-1197.

end-stage patients in palliative care.[16] The therapeutic effects appear to be both rapid and sustained, lasting for several months or even years after treatment.

While direct research on the effects of psilocybin on insomnia is limited, there is evidence suggesting that psilocybin may indirectly help manage insomnia by alleviating anxiety and depression, which are often associated with sleep disturbances.[17] Several studies have investigated the potential therapeutic benefits of psilocybin for mental health issues.

While these studies do not focus specifically on insomnia, they demonstrate psilocybin's potential to address anxiety and depression, which can contribute to sleep disturbances. Further research is needed to establish the efficacy of psilocybin in managing insomnia directly. However, these studies provide a foundation for understanding its potential therapeutic effects on related mental health issues.

---

16 Reiche, S., Hermle, L., Gutwinski, S., et al. (2018). Serotonergic hallucinogens in the treatment of anxiety and depression in patients suffering from a life-threatening disease: A systematic review. Progress in Neuro-Psychopharmacology and Biological Psychiatry, 81, 1-10.

17 Riemann, D., & Voderholzer, U. (2003). Primary insomnia: a risk factor to develop depression? Journal of Affective Disorders, 76(1-3), 255-259.

THE FUTURE OF PSYCHEDELIC HEALTH CARE

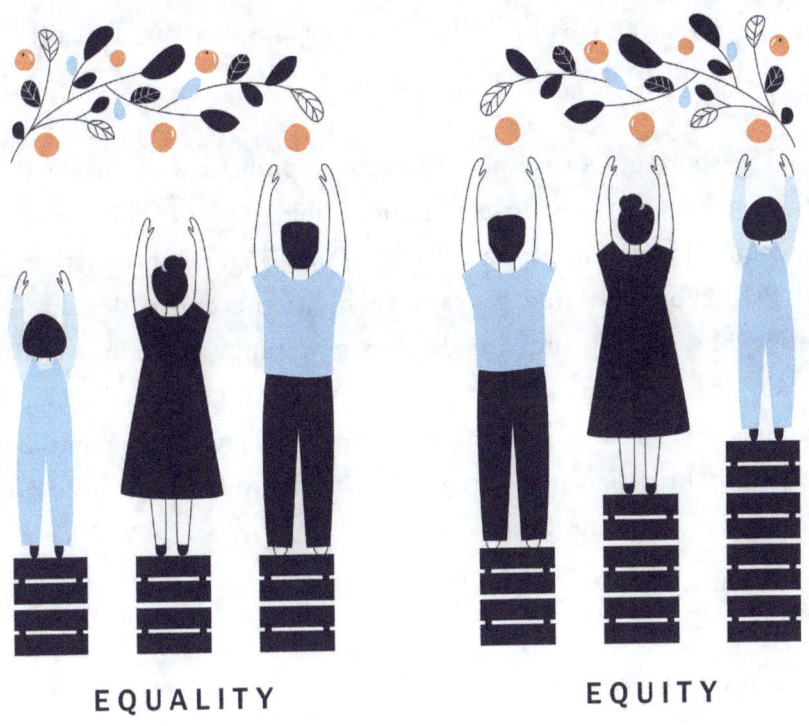

EQUALITY EQUITY

According to the American Psychological Association, the United States is facing a shortage of therapists. By 2032, the country is projected to need twice as many therapists as it currently has.

This shortage is caused by a number of factors, including:

- The Baby Boomer generation is aging, and many members are experiencing mental health problems such as anxiety and depression.
- The rising cost of healthcare is making it more difficult for people to afford therapy.

The shortage of therapists is a serious problem, as it means that many people who need help will not be able to get it. This can have a negative impact on people's health, well-being, and productivity.

Psilocybin-assisted therapy involves the controlled use of psilocybin, to help individuals manage a range of mental health conditions. This type of therapy typically involves a trained therapist administering a carefully measured dose of psilocybin in a controlled setting, while also providing emotional support and guidance throughout the experience.

CHAPTER 1

Psilocybin "Magic" Mushrooms

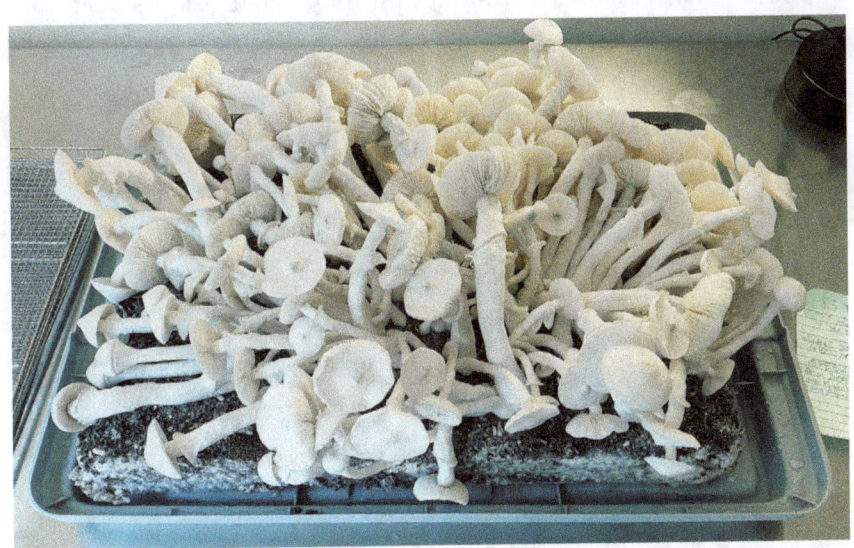

This is the second flush of fresh Albino Avery to be harvested and then dried. Mushrooms are grown in covered tubs and conditions which imitate the humid Amazonian climate.

Psilocybin mushrooms are a type of psychedelic fungus that contain psychoactive compounds such as psilocybin and psilocin. They are also known as "magic mushrooms", "'shrooms", "boomers", "fungus", and "mushies." They have been used for thousands of years in various cultures around the world for their powerful effects on consciousness.

The earliest documented use of magic mushrooms dates back to the pre-Columbian era in Mesoamerica, where they were used for their psychoactive effects in religious and spiritual ceremonies. The Aztecs referred to them as teonanácatl, which translates to "flesh of the gods." There is also evidence of their use in indigenous cultures in South America. They can induce profound changes in perception, emotions, cognition, mood, and thought, and the acute effects can last several hours.

Psilocybin mushrooms grow wild just about everywhere, yet they are illegal to grow, possess or consume in many countries, including the United States, where they are classified as a Schedule I controlled substance. This means that they are considered to have a high potential for abuse and no accepted medical use.

Decriminalization has been an instrumental first step in orienting people to psilocybin by removing the fear of criminal prosecution for possession and use of the substance. Decriminalization efforts have been successful in several cities and states in the United States, and in countries like Jamaica, where psilocybin mushrooms are legal and decriminalized. This has allowed for a shift in public perception towards psilocybin, from a dangerous and illegal drug to a potentially beneficial substance that can be used for personal development and spiritual growth. Decriminalization has also opened up opportunities for research into the therapeutic potential of psilocybin, as researchers no longer have to worry about legal barriers to studying the substance. This has led to a growing body of scientific evidence supporting the use of psilocybin in treating mental health disorders such as depression, anxiety, and PTSD. Furthermore, decriminalization has allowed for the emergence of a community of people who are interested in exploring the potential benefits of psilocybin in a safe and responsible manner. This community includes advocates, researchers, therapists, and individuals who use psilocybin for personal development and spiritual growth. By removing the fear of criminal prosecution, decriminalization has helped to foster a more open and accepting attitude towards psilocybin, which has in turn led to increased interest in its potential benefits.

Psilocybin mushrooms should be approached with caution despite their numerous benefits. Always be aware of the potential risks, such as adverse reactions or unwanted psychological effects. If you have a history of mental illness or are currently taking medications, consult with a professional facilitator or therapist before embarking on this journey.

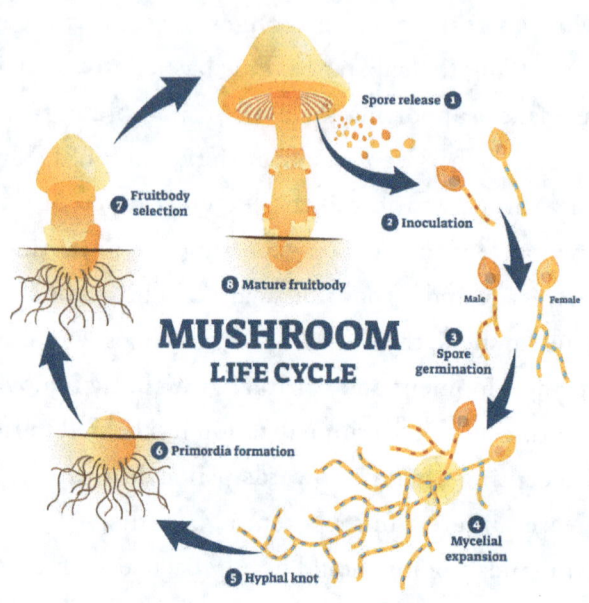

The lifecycle of a magic mushroom, or *Psilocybe Cubensis*, begins with spores released from mature fruiting bodies. These microscopic spores land on a suitable substrate, such as decaying plant material or dung, and germinate, producing thread-like structures called mycelium. The mycelium grows, colonizing the substrate, and eventually forms a dense network. Under the right environmental conditions—typically, high humidity and cooler temperatures—the mycelium starts to produce fruiting bodies. The fruiting bodies, or mushrooms, emerge from the mycelium as small pins, which then grow. Once mature, the they release their spores, thus completing the lifecycle and starting a new generation.

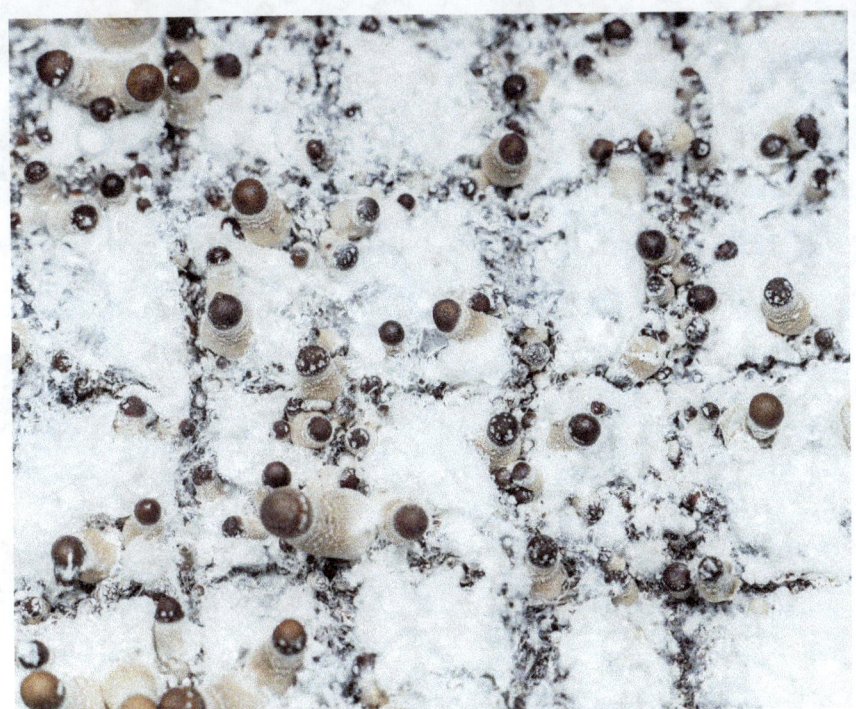

Tiny mushroom 'pins' popping out of the substrate.

The time it takes to complete the entire lifecycle of a magic mushroom can vary depending on factors such as species, environmental conditions, and the type of substrate used. Generally, it takes about four to six weeks from the initial spore germination to fruiting body maturity. The mycelium typically colonizes the substrate within two to three weeks, while the fruiting and maturation of mushrooms can take another two to three weeks. It's important to note that these timelines can be shorter or longer, depending on specific environmental conditions and the strain of mushroom used.

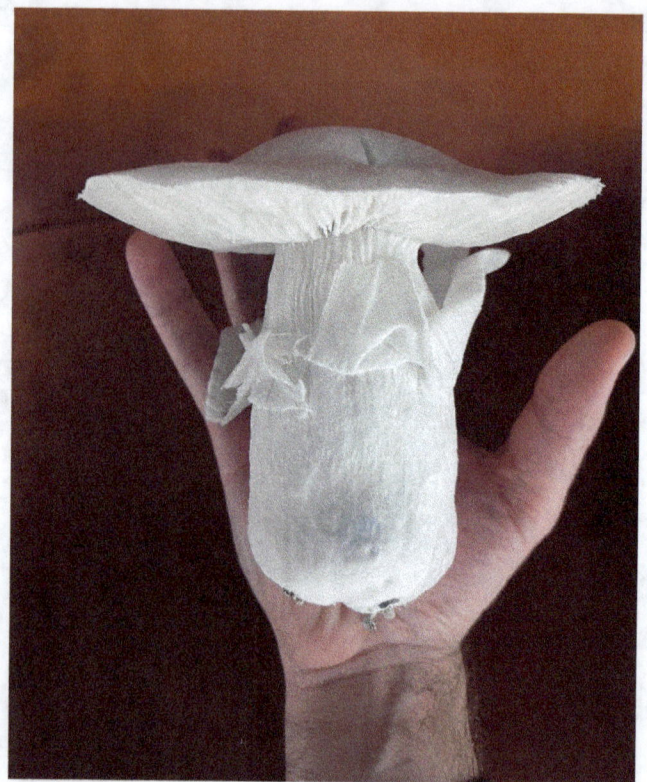

This is a giant Psilocybe Cubensis Albino Penis Envy 221 specimen that weighs over 50g fresh and lacks any pigment.

Magic mushrooms are made of *Chitin*, a complex polysaccharide compound that makes up a significant portion of the cell walls in fungi, including fruiting bodies. It is composed of long chains of a nitrogen-containing sugar called N-acetylglucosamine, which is linked together by chemical bonds. Chitin is responsible for providing structural support and rigidity to the cell walls of mushrooms, helping to maintain their shape and protect them from external stressors. Chitin is also a major component of the exoskeletons of insects and other arthropods, as well as the shells of crustaceans such as crabs and lobsters. It's believed to cause the nausea that sometimes occurs when a Seeker consumes high doses of magic mushrooms, but more research is needed.

Magic mushrooms can be consumed in a variety of ways, including eaten raw or dried, steeped into tea, taken in capsules filled with dried mushrooms or psilocybin extract, microdosed, or in the form of psilocybin-infused edibles. It's important to note that the dosage and method of consumption can greatly impact the effects of magic mushrooms' psychoactive ingredients, and it's always important to take caution and follow harm reduction guidelines when using any of these techniques.

Magic mushrooms are considered hydrophilic (water-loving) because they contain a high amount of water-soluble compounds, such as psilocybin and psilocin, which are responsible for their psychoactive effects. These compounds have a strong affinity for water molecules and are readily dissolved in water or other polar solvents. In fact, water is often used as a medium to extract active psilocybin into tea for use in various forms of therapy and research. The hydrophilic nature of magic mushrooms also means that they can easily absorb water and other substances from their environment, which can be a concern when it comes to environmental contaminants and potential toxicity.

Dosages and effects vary depending on the Seeker's physiology as well. Factors such as low stomach acid may impact the absorption and effectiveness of psilocybin mushrooms. Stomach acid plays a role in breaking down food and releasing various compounds, including psilocybin, from the ingested mushrooms. Some individuals have a slower digestive process, which could lead to a decreased release of psilocybin and potentially affect its conversion to psilocin[18].

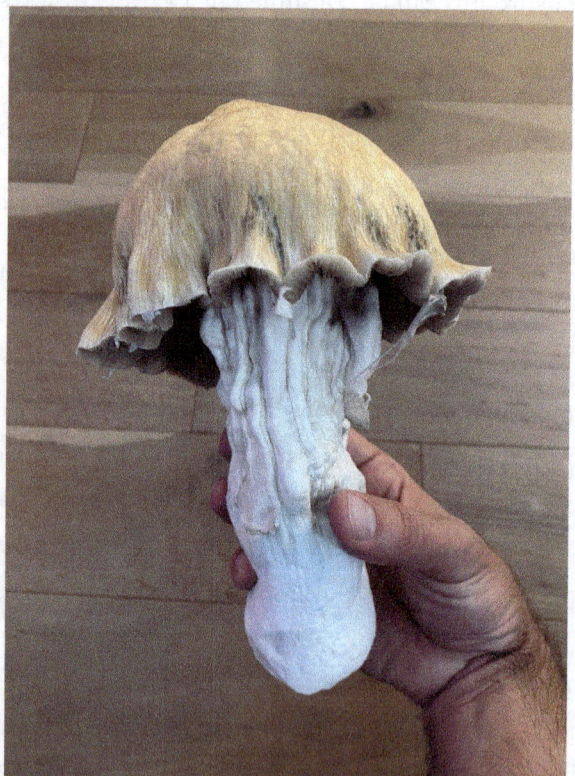

Fresh Psilocybe Cubensis Great Golden Monster

---

18 Turek, F.W., & Gillette, M.U., "Melatonin, sleep, and circadian rhythms: rationale for development of specific melatonin agonists," Sleep Medicine, 2004, https://www.sciencedirect.com/science/article/abs/pii/S1389945704001819.

Another issue that may arise from low stomach acid is the increased risk of rapid oxidation. Oxidation can occur when compounds are exposed to oxygen and reactive molecules, resulting in a loss of potency[19]. In the cases of psilocybin and psilocin, if their release and conversion are slowed down due to low stomach acid, they may remain in the gastrointestinal tract for a longer period, increasing the likelihood of oxidation. This is why it's recommended that you take mushrooms with antioxidants.

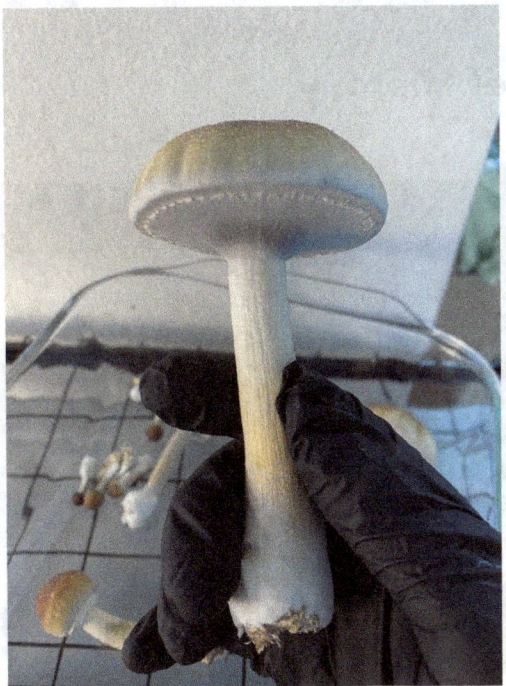

Fresh Psilocybe Cubensis Burma

19 Zhang, A., Sun, H., & Wang, X., "Recent advances in natural products from plants for treatment of liver diseases," European Journal of Medicinal Chemistry, 2013, https://www.sciencedirect.com/science/article/abs/pii/S0223523412006702.

As a result, individuals with low stomach acid may experience diminished or inconsistent effects from psilocybin-containing mushrooms. It is worth noting that various factors can influence the absorption, metabolism, and effects of psilocybin, including individual differences in genetics, metabolism, and gut microbiota[20]. Therefore, the effects of low stomach acid on psilocybin's efficacy may vary among individuals.

1.1 A Brief History

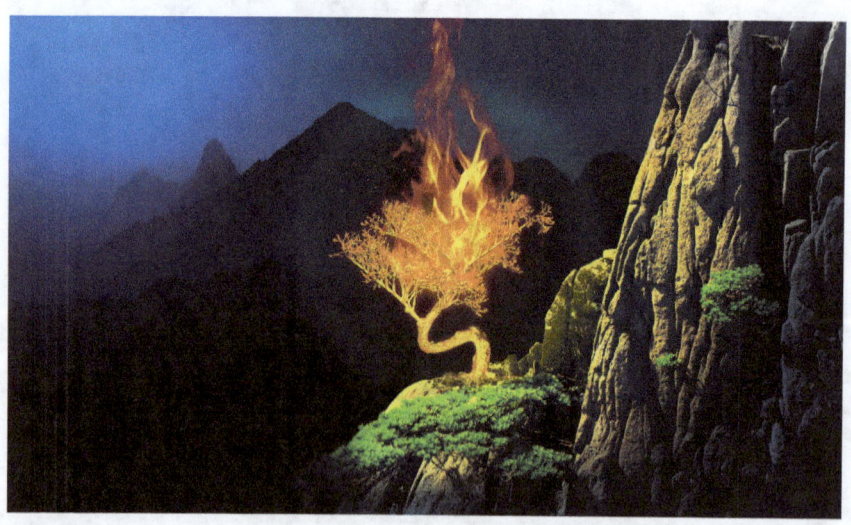

---

20 Dinan, T.G., & Cryan, J.F., "The Microbiome-Gut-Brain Axis in Health and Disease," Gastroenterology Clinics of North America, 2017, https://www.sciencedirect.com/science/article/abs/pii/S0889855316300826.

Throughout history, entheogens—psychoactive substances used for spiritual or religious purposes. There are even suggestions that the Bible contains references to entheogenic substances. Some scholars propose that certain passages, such as the description of the Tree of Knowledge of Good and Evil in Genesis or the visionary experiences of the prophets, may allude to the use of entheogens, including Psilocybin mushrooms.

Timothy Leary, a Harvard psychologist, and Richard Alpert, who later became known as Ram Dass, conducted the Harvard Psilocybin Project, further drawing attention to the substance. Terence McKenna, an ethnobotanist and philosopher, contributed to the popularization of magic mushrooms through his books, lectures, and advocacy for the exploration of altered states of consciousness using psychedelic substances.

Paul Stamets, a renowned mycologist and author and Jeff Chilton, a pioneer in the cultivation of medicinal mushrooms, have been instrumental in advancing the understanding of psilocybin mushrooms, their cultivation, and potential therapeutic uses. They played an essential role in promoting the use of magic mushrooms for both their psychoactive and therapeutic properties in their book "The Mushroom Cultivator: A Practical Guide to Growing Mushrooms at Home."

One of the most notable figures in the history of Psilocybin mushrooms is Maria Sabina, a Mazatec *curandera* (healer) from Mexico. Born in the early 1900s, Maria Sabina grew up in the small village of Huautla de Jiménez in the Sierra Mazateca of

Oaxaca, Mexico. She was introduced to the ceremonial use of Psilocybin mushrooms at a young age and became a *curandera* in her community.

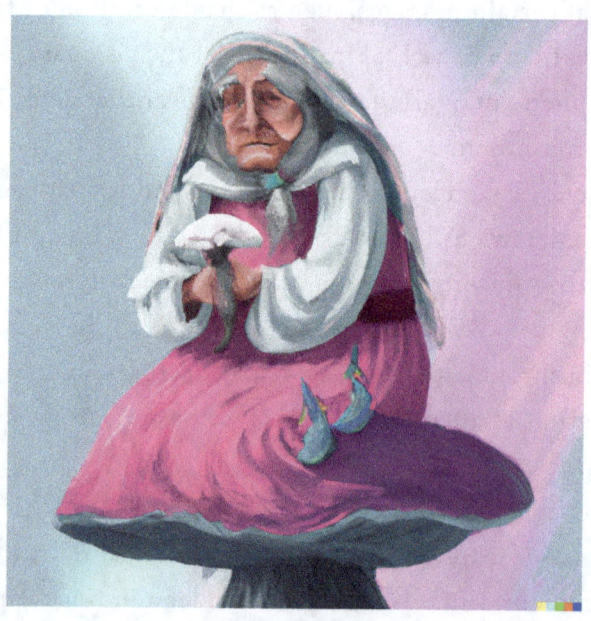

In the 1950s, Maria Sabina's life took a dramatic turn when R. Gordon Wasson, an American ethnomycologist, and his wife, Valentina, visited her to learn about and participate in a traditional mushroom ceremony.

Among the Mazatec indigenous people of Mexico, the psychoactive substances contained in the psilocybe mushrooms are known as "Teonanacatl," which translates to "God's flesh" in the Aztec language. Teonanacatl is considered a sacred substance used in the context of religious ceremonies and is believed to facilitate communication with spirits and divinities.

The Wassons' experience with Maria Sabina eventually led to an article in *Life* magazine, which introduced Psilocybin mushrooms to a global audience.

As a result of this publicity, Maria Sabina's village was inundated with outsiders seeking the powerful effects of the mushrooms that the article described. Unfortunately, this attention had severe consequences for Maria Sabina and her community. She faced ostracism from her fellow villagers, who believed that she had desecrated their sacred traditions. Additionally, the Mexican government cracked down on the use of Psilocybin mushrooms, further complicating the situation for Maria Sabina and her people by restricted their cultivation and use in ceremony.

Psilocybin was banned in the United States and listed as a Schedule I controlled substance mainly due to its potential for recreational abuse and no recognized medical uses at that time, as well as its belief as a "mind-altering drug" that could be a potential danger to public safety and health. The law was also influenced by the broader social and cultural movements during the time, such as the Vietnam War, counterculture, and youth rebellion, which psychedelics were associated with. The banning of psilocybin and other psychedelics occurred after the widespread media attention on Timothy Leary's advocacy, who believed that the substances could enhance personal growth, spirituality, and social change, which was viewed as a threat to the established political and social norms of the time.

This connection led to negative perceptions and fears among some segments of society, and drugs—especially psychedelics—began to be viewed as dangerous and destabilizing. The recent legalization push for the use of psilocybin and other psychedelics, especially in the field of medicine, is because of the ongoing scientific research and evidence that indicates their potential to treat mental health disorders such as anxiety, depression, PTSD, and addiction. After several decades of criminalization and neglect, researchers and advocates are rediscovering the therapeutic benefits and potential of psychedelics, which is opening new avenues for treatments beyond the traditional methods. Additionally, the cultural stigma towards these substances is gradually declining, and they are starting to be viewed in a more positive light. This shift in attitudes is reflected in the recent widespread decriminalization trends in various cities, states, and countries, which are trying to create more comprehensive regulatory frameworks for their responsible use. Furthermore, the recent legalization push is in line with the changing political landscapes and public opinion towards drug reform, especially towards drug policies that take a public health approach rather than a punitive one.

The culmination of these factors eventually led to the passage of the Controlled Substances Act of 1970, which classified psilocybin as a Schedule I substance, along with other drugs like LSD, marijuana[21], and heroin. Schedule I drugs were defined as having a high potential for abuse, no accepted medical use, and a lack of safety for use under medical supervision.

---

21 *Marijuana* is DEA terminology—the correct term is *Cannabis*.

1.2 Mushrooms Fruiting-Bodies

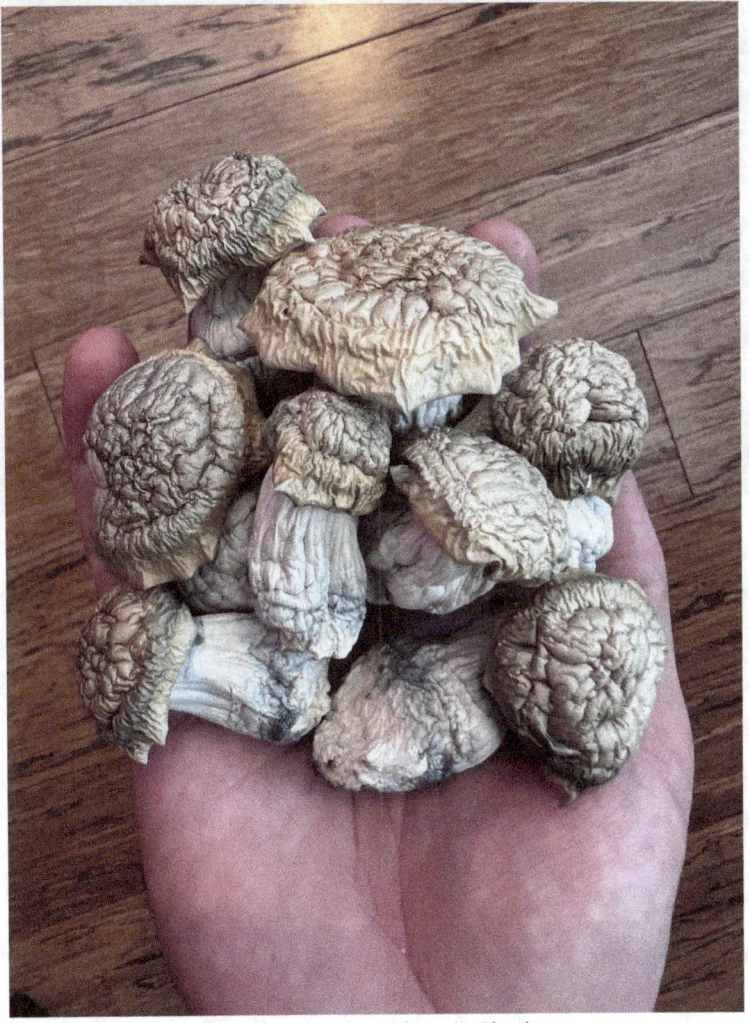

Dried Psilocybe Cubensis Choda

The fruiting body of magic mushrooms, often referred to as the mushroom cap, is the visible part of the mushroom that grows above ground and contains the spores responsible for reproduction. The fruiting body comes in various colors, shapes, and sizes, depending on the species, environment, and growing conditions. The cap is mostly convex, conical, or umbonate, with a central nipple-like structure called the umbo. The texture of the cap surface can range from smooth to wavy, and it may or may not have a veil or partial veil structure. Under the cap, there are thin gills that radiate outward from the stem, which produces the spores once the mushroom reaches maturity. The color of the gills can vary from white to purple or brown, depending on the species. The stem of magic mushrooms can range from thin and fragile to thick and robust, and it can be hollow or solid. The stem's color can vary from white to yellow, brown, or blue, depending on the species and environmental factors such as light exposure or bruising. Overall, the external characteristics of magic mushroom fruiting bodies are important for their identification and classification, as well as for their potential medicinal and recreational uses.

If you see blue or green stains on the mushrooms, don't worry. That's just the result of oxidized psilocin, and can occur when the mushrooms are mishandled. It's easy to confuse bruising for mold.

Look for mushrooms with healthy, well-formed caps and stems. They should not appear slimy, discolored, or moldy.

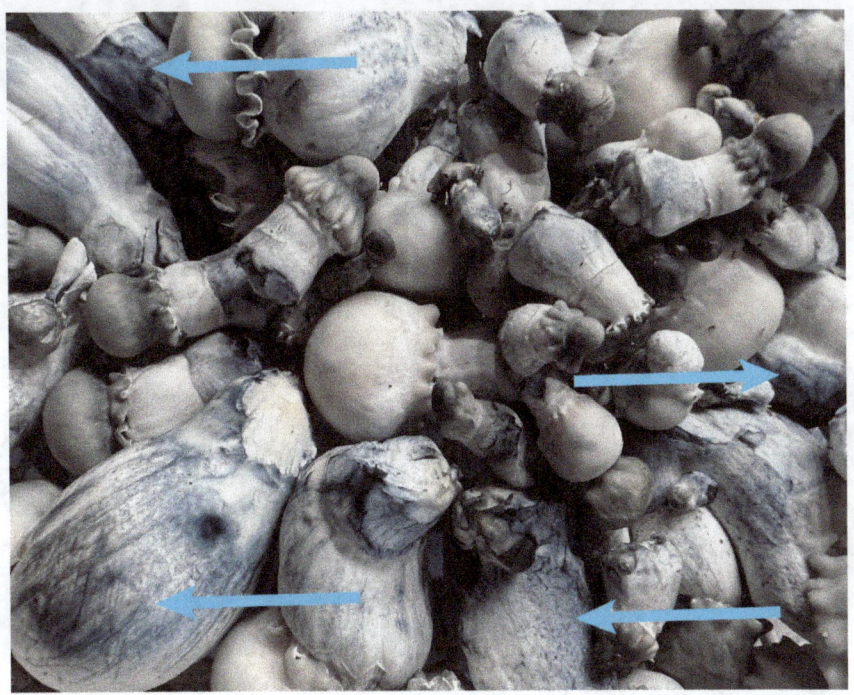

Blue or light green patches are not mold but often oxidized psilocin, which is safe to consume.

Signs of contamination:

- Off smell: A strong, unpleasant odor that deviates from the typical earthy smell of mushrooms.
- Sliminess: A slimy texture on the mushroom surface may suggest bacterial contamination.
- Foreign materials: Presence of contaminants such as dark spores, vermiculite, coir, compost, or hair.

1.2.1 Foraged Mushrooms

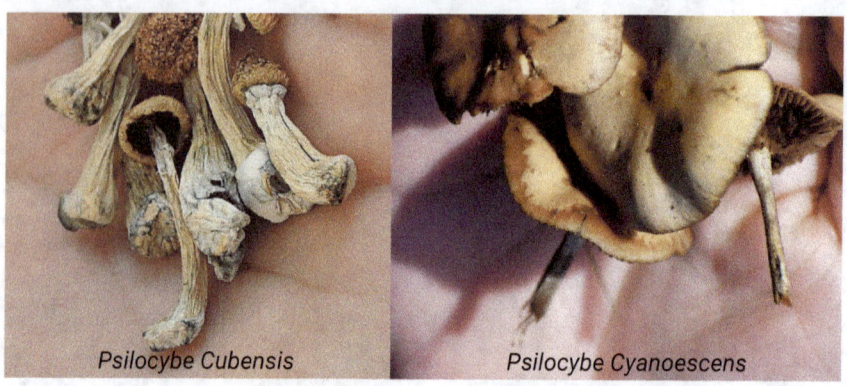

Psilocybe Cubensis   *Psilocybe Cyanoescens*

There are many strains of magic mushrooms, including *Psilocybe cubensis*, the most common, and *Psilocybe semilanceata*, *Psilocybe mexicana*, *Psilocybe azurescens*, and *Psilocybe cyanescens*. Each has its own unique properties and effects.

There are several species of mushrooms that can be mistaken for magic mushrooms, including *Panaeolus cinctulus*, *Gymnopilus junonius*, *Psathyrella candolleana*, and *Galerina marginata*. It's important to note that if you are not an experienced mycologist, it can be difficult to accurately identify mushrooms in the wild.

It's always best to err on the side of caution and only consume lab-grown mushrooms because identifying wild mushrooms can be a risky and complicated process, particularly for those without expert knowledge. Many wild mushroom species contain toxins that can cause severe and even life-threatening symptoms such as nausea, vomiting, diarrhea, abdominal pain, liver damage, kidney failure, hallucinations, and even death. It can be challenging to differentiate between edible and poisonous mushrooms based on their appearances alone, as many poisonous species closely resemble edible ones. Therefore, it is essential to have a professional mushroom specialist identify the species before consuming or avoiding them. By consuming lab-grown mushrooms, you can be sure that the mushrooms are safe, free from toxins, and their cultivation process is controlled and regulated. Additionally, lab-grown mushrooms are often of high quality, potency, and purity, making them ideal for medicinal and recreational use. Therefore, it is always best to err on the side of caution and consume lab-grown mushrooms, particularly for those who are not experts in mushroom identification.

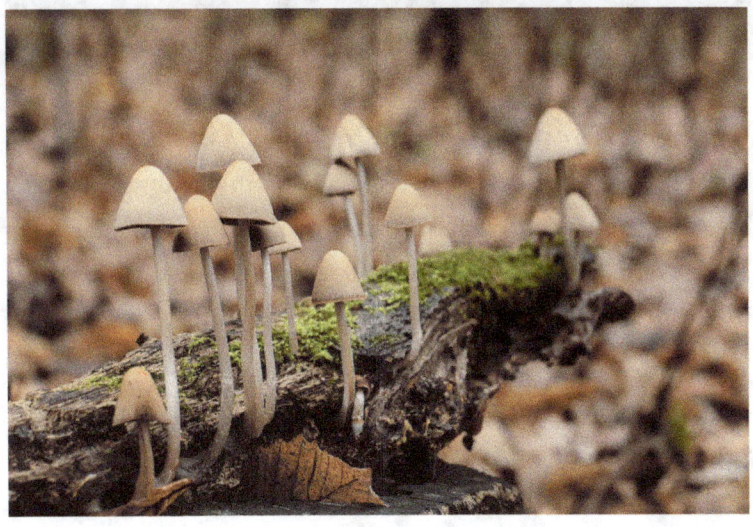

Panaeolus cinctulus mushrooms, also known as the blue ring mushroom, contain toxins that can cause symptoms such as nausea, vomiting, cramps, and diarrhea. In rare cases, consumption can lead to liver and kidney damage, and even death.

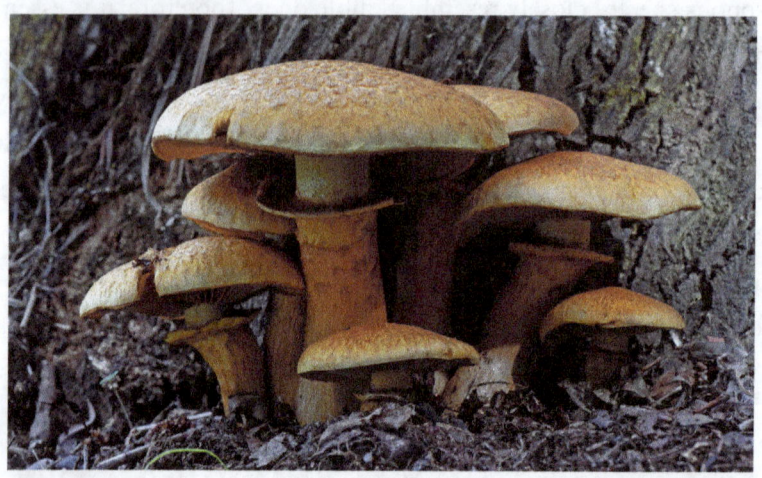

Gymnopilus junonius, commonly known as Laughing Gym or Big Laughing Gym, is a species of mushroom that can be easily confused with Psilocybe cubensis, also known as Magic Mushroom. The two species share some similarities in their physical appearance, which can make it difficult to differentiate between them. Both species produce a cap with a broad, convex shape and a firm texture. The most apparent difference between the two is that G. junonius does not contain psychoactive compounds like psilocybin and psilocin, while P. cubensis produces these compounds, which are responsible for the hallucinogenic effects. Therefore, it is essential to be cautious when hunting for wild mushrooms and to have a qualified expert identify any species of mushroom before consumption, particularly if you are new to mushroom identification.

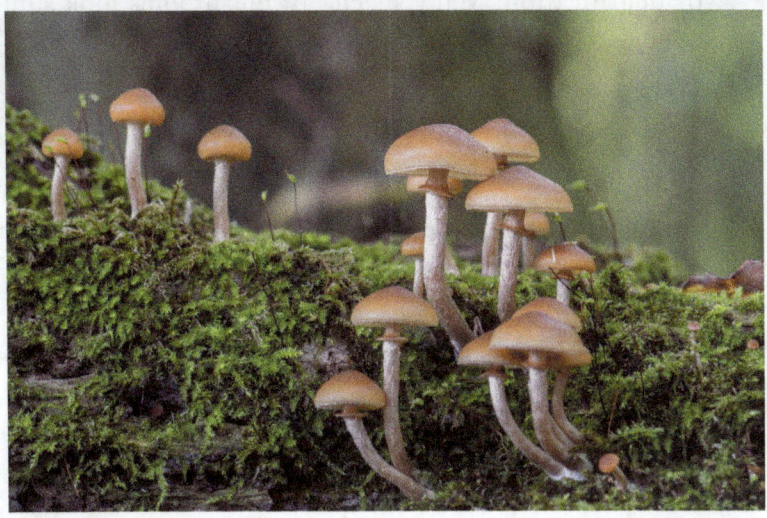

Galerina marginata mushrooms, also known as "deadly galerina" or "autumn skullcap," contain the toxin amatoxins. Amatoxins interfere with protein synthesis in the liver and can cause irreversible liver damage or even death if ingested. Symptoms of poisoning may not appear for several hours or even days after ingestion and can include nausea, vomiting, abdominal pain, diarrhea, and yellowing of the skin and eyes (jaundice). *Galerina marginata* mushrooms are often mistaken for edible varieties and are responsible for a number of poisonings and fatalities each year.

Foraging mushrooms in the wild can be risky due to several factors:

- Misidentification: Many species of mushrooms look similar, and it can be challenging to differentiate between psychoactive and toxic varieties. Consuming toxic mushrooms can result in severe poisoning or even death.
- Environmental contaminants: Wild mushrooms may be exposed to pesticides, pollutants, or other toxic substances, which can be harmful when ingested.

1.2.2 Lab-Grown Mushrooms

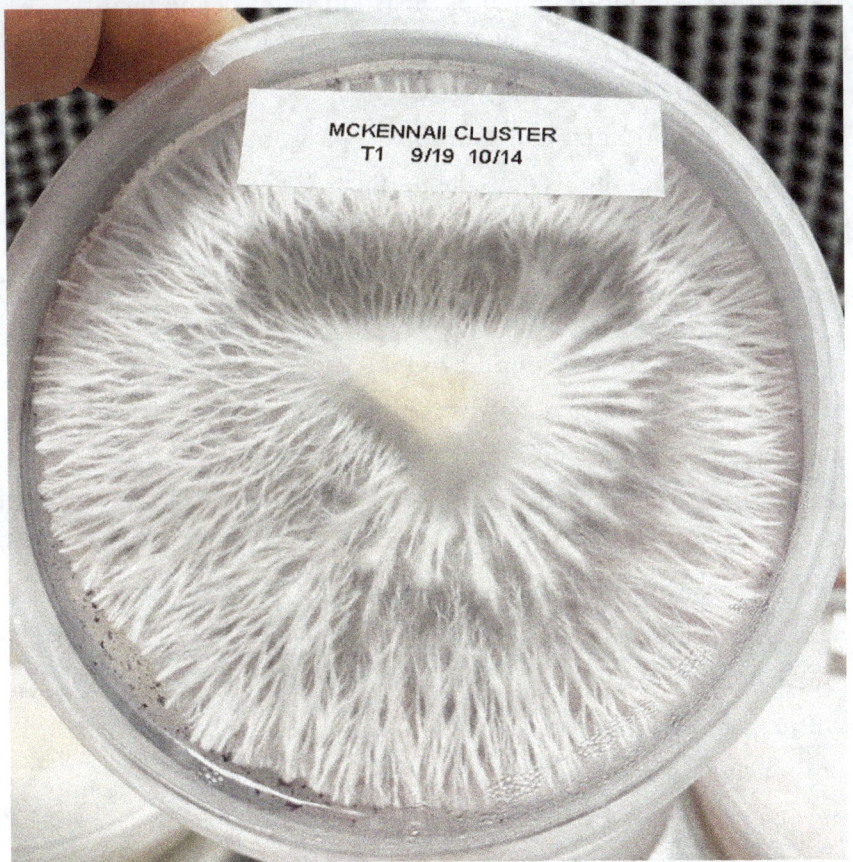

Tissue cultured P. Cubensis McKennaii growing Rhizomorphic mycelium on an agar plate.

Lab-grown or cultivated mushrooms can provide a safer alternative to foraged mushrooms because they can be grown in sterile, controlled environments, minimizing the risk of misidentification and contamination. Additionally, the cultivation process can be standardized, resulting in more consistent potency and quality.

1.2.3 Counterfeit Products

The underground magic mushroom market is a growing industry, and with it comes the risk of fake products. These products are those that are made to look like genuine products but are of inferior quality or contain harmful ingredients. In the case of magic mushrooms, counterfeit products can pose a serious food safety risk.

Psychedelic underground products, such as those sold on the black market or online, are often of unknown origin, purity, and potency, and can pose significant health risks to consumers. Some common types of these products that are sold on underground markets include LSD, psilocybin mushrooms, DMT, and other synthetic or natural psychoactive substances. An analysis of these products has shown that they often contain other compounds in addition to the primary active ingredient.

In addition to containing harmful chemicals, counterfeit magic mushroom products can

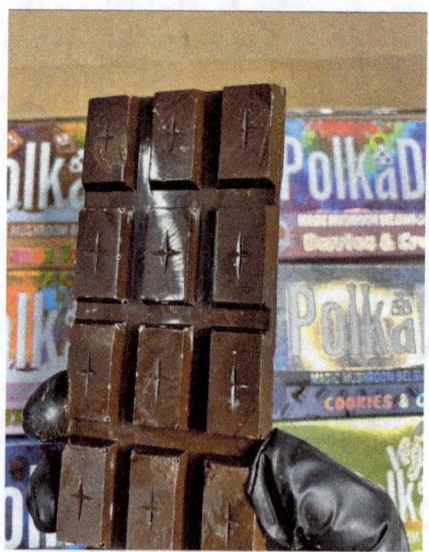

Polkadot is an online brand with at least 2 instagram pages that compete with one another. Old rivalries perhaps?

also be mislabeled. This means that the product may not contain the amount of psilocybin or other psychoactive compounds that it is advertised to contain. This can lead to Seekers taking more of the product than they intended, which can increase the risk of negative side effects.

One such example is the One Up brand, which sells fake packaging alongside a chocolate-making kit, allowing anyone with a few dollars to deceive the public to appear as an authentic edible brand.

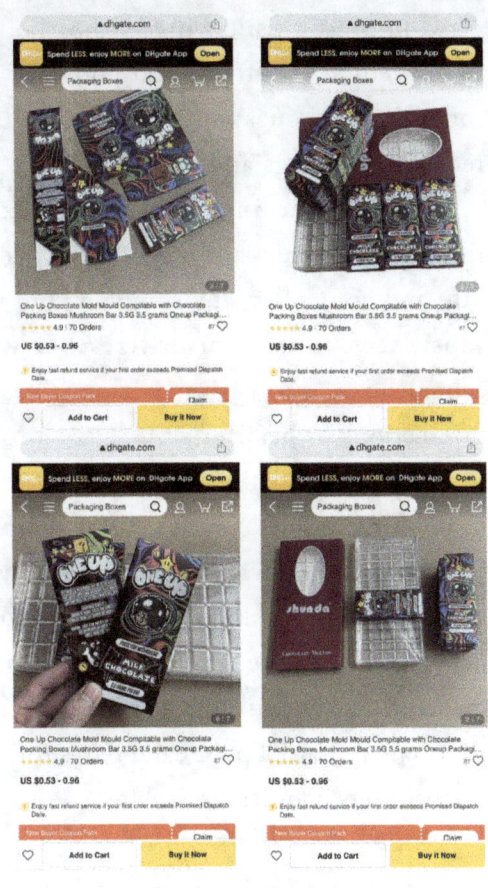

Here is an example of a OneUp kit on DHGate, a Chinese marketplace. Reddit is a good place to research sources.

1.2.4 Possible Interactions

Psilocybin mushrooms have been shown to be relatively safe when used responsibly, but there are certain contraindications and risk factors that should be considered before using them.

Combining psilocybin with other recreational drugs can lead to unpredictable effects and potential risks. This section addresses some common questions people have about the interactions between recreational drugs and psilocybin.

While some individuals may experiment with combining recreational drugs and psilocybin, it's generally best to do so in a safe and controlled environment, and without also ingesting other substances. Always prioritize your well-being and consult with a healthcare professional if you have concerns about potential interactions or health risks.

A contraindication which refers to a specific situation, symptom, or medical condition that makes a particular treatment, medication, or procedure inadvisable or potentially harmful for a patient. This means that the risks of a particular treatment may outweigh the benefits or that the treatment may negatively interact with another medication or condition that a person has.

Some potential poor candidates for Psilocybin use include people with serious conditions such as:

1. *Mental health disorders*: Individuals with a personal or family history of schizophrenia, psychosis, bipolar disorder, or other severe mental health conditions should avoid using Psilocybin, as it may exacerbate these conditions or trigger the onset of symptoms.
2. *Anxiety disorders*: People with deep trauma, anxiety disorders or a predisposition to anxiety may be more susceptible to experiencing

increased panic or paranoia during a high-dose Psilocybin experience.

3. *Heart conditions*: Psilocybin can cause slight increases in heart rate and blood pressure, which may pose risks for individuals with pre-existing heart conditions or cardiovascular issues.

4. *Seizure disorders*: Although it is not common, Psilocybin could induce further seizures in individuals with a history of epilepsy or seizure disorders.

5. *Pregnancy and breastfeeding*: The effects of Psilocybin on pregnant or breastfeeding individuals and their infants have not been well-studied. It is generally advised to avoid using Psilocybin during pregnancy and breastfeeding to ensure the safety of both mother and child.

1.2.4.1 Alcohol

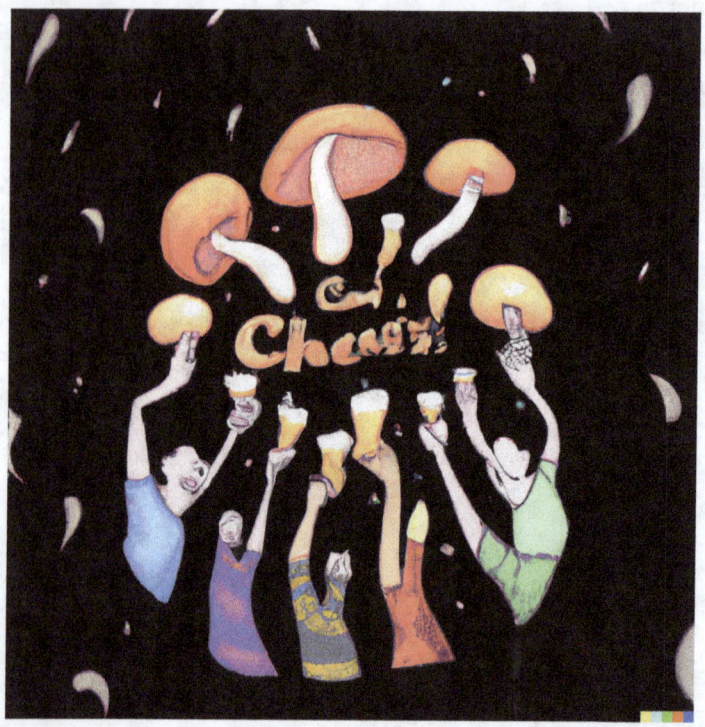

Mixing psilocybin and alcohol is generally not recommended, as alcohol can dull the effects of psilocybin and potentially lead to nausea, vomiting, or increased disorientation. Combining these substances can also exacerbate negative emotions and anxiety, potentially resulting in an unpleasant experience.

In a 2010 study led by David Nutt, psilocybin was found to be the least toxic substance when compared to the twenty most commonly used drugs[22] while alcohol was the most harmful. While alcohol is a legal and socially accepted substance in America, it is associated with numerous health and social issues. This study evaluated these drugs based on multiple factors, including physical harm, dependence potential, and social harm.

According to the National Institute on Alcohol Abuse and Alcoholism (NIAAA), approximately 95,000 deaths are attributed to excessive alcohol use[23] in the United States each year. Alcohol consumption has been linked to various health issues, such as liver disease, cardiovascular problems, and cancer. Additionally, alcohol use has been connected to an increased risk of depression and anxiety, exacerbating existing mental health conditions or contributing to new ones.[24] Alcohol use also tends to significantly impact social problems like domestic violence, traffic accidents, and criminal behavior.

In contrast, Psilocybin has been found to have a relatively low potential for harm, with fewer adverse health effects and a lower risk for dependence.[25] Psilocybin is considered to have a favorable safety

---

22 Nutt, D., King, L.A., & Phillips, L.D., "Drug harms in the UK: a multicriteria decision analysis," The Lancet, 2010, https://www.thelancet.com/journals/lancet/article/PIIS0140-6736(10)61462-6/fulltext.

23 NIAAA, "Alcohol Facts and Statistics," https://www.niaaa.nih.gov/publications/brochures-and-fact-sheets/alcohol-facts-and-statistics.

24 World Health Organization, "Alcohol," https://www.who.int/news-room/fact-sheets/detail/alcohol.

25 Nutt, D. J., King, L. A., & Phillips, L. D. (2010). Drug harms in the UK: a multicriteria decision analysis. The Lancet, 376(9752), 1558-1565.

profile, and while it is not without risk, the associated dangers of its use are significantly lower than those of alcohol and other drugs.[26]

It is essential, however, to emphasize the importance of responsible use and proper preparation, guidance, and integration in psychedelic experiences to minimize potential harm. Safety issues associated with psilocybin rarely stem from the physical substance itself. Lack of research, awareness, and integration are often the leading causes of any negative outcomes.

1.2.4.3 Cannabis

The effects of combining psilocybin and cannabis can be unpredictable, as both substances have psychoactive properties. Some Seekers report enhanced visuals and a more intensity, while others may experience increased anxiety, paranoia, or confusion. It's important to be cautious when combining these substances and to consider factors such as individual sensitivity, tolerance, and dosage.

1.2.4.4 Stimulants

Combining psilocybin with stimulants is generally not recommended, as this can lead to increased heart rate, blood pressure, and anxiety. The stimulating effects of substances like Adderall, cocaine, or other amphetamines may clash with the introspective nature of a psilocybin experience, potentially resulting in an uncomfortable or distressing "trip."

---

26 Dos Santos, R. G., Osório, F. L., Crippa, J. A. S., Riba, J., Zuardi, A. W., & Hallak, J. E. C. (2016). Antidepressive, anxiolytic, and antiaddictive effects of ayahuasca, Psilocybin and lysergic acid diethylamide (LSD): a systematic review of clinical trials published in the peer-reviewed scientific literature.

1.2.4.5 MDMA (Ecstasy)

The combination of psilocybin and MDMA is sometimes referred to as a "hippie flip." While some Seekers report euphoric and synergistic effects, others may experience intensified emotions, anxiety, or confusion. This particular combination can also put increased strain on the cardiovascular system. It's essential to approach this specific pairing with caution and to consider factors such as dosage, individual sensitivity, and the setting in which the substances are consumed.

1.2.4.6 SSRIs / Antidepressants

If someone is currently taking selective serotonin reuptake inhibitors (SSRIs) for a mental health condition, it is generally recommended that they speak with their healthcare provider before stopping the medication. Abruptly stopping SSRIs can lead to withdrawal symptoms, which may include nausea, headache, dizziness, insomnia, and anxiety. Therefore, it is important to slowly taper off the medication under the supervision of a healthcare provider if one is considering getting off SSRIs. In terms of taking psilocybin, there is limited research on combining psilocybin with SSRIs.

While some individuals have safely combined the two, it is important to understand that SSRIs can alter the effects of psilocybin and may reduce the intensity of the psychedelic experience or interact in unpredictable ways, which might be undesirable if one is seeking the full therapeutic potential of psilocybin. For this reason, some researchers suggest that individuals considering taking psilocybin for therapeutic purposes may benefit from stopping their use of SSRIs temporarily before taking psilocybin. However, this decision should be made in consultation with their healthcare provider, since the benefits and risks of stopping or reducing antidepressants vary for each individual. Overall, it is essential that individuals considering taking psilocybin for medical purposes discuss their medical history, including their use of SSRIs, with a healthcare provider before deciding to take psilocybin. The healthcare provider can help guide the decision-making process and minimize risks for the individual.

If someone is currently taking monoamine oxidase inhibitors (MAOIs), they should exercise caution before taking psilocybin. MAOIs are commonly prescribed for depression, but they can interact with psilocybin with potentially dangerous side effects. The combination of MAOIs and psilocybin can increase the levels of serotonin in the brain to dangerous levels. This can lead to serotonin syndrome, which could cause symptoms ranging from mild, such as shivering and diarrhea, to severe, such as muscle rigidity, fever, and seizures. Severe serotonin syndrome can cause death if not treated. Therefore, it is recommended that individuals should taper off and discontinue MAOIs for at least two weeks before taking psilocybin. If one decides to take psilocybin without tapering off MAOIs, they may want to use a smaller dose. Nevertheless, it is important to speak with a healthcare provider before making any changes to medication regimes. Individuals who are considering taking psilocybin and who are currently taking MAOIs should speak with a healthcare provider before doing so. The healthcare provider can help guide the decision-making process and minimize risks of adverse reactions such as serotonin syndrome.

Getting off SSRIs and MAOIs can be a challenging process, so taper off slowly and reduce the dose gradually under the guidance of a healthcare provider. Abruptly stopping SSRIs can lead to withdrawal symptoms such as dizziness, nausea, and anxiety, so it is important to be patient and take things slowly. It may take several weeks or months to taper off completely. If one experiences any discomfort during the process, they are advised to talk to their healthcare provider. It is important to remember that getting off SSRIs is a process that takes time and patience.

1.2.5 Synergistic Compounds

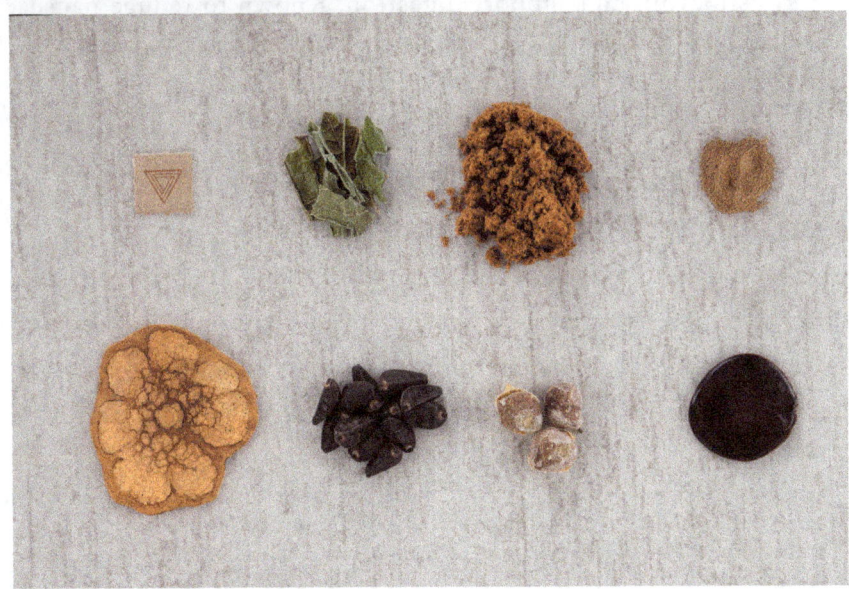

(GI) discomfort are common issues that individuals may experience when consuming magic mushrooms. This is because Psilocybin can irritate the stomach lining and cause contractions in the GI tract. Some remedies that may help alleviate nausea and GI issues include consuming the mushrooms with ginger, taking antacids, and eating a light meal before.

How to improve the culinary experience:

- *Acidic Activator*: Enhances the absorption of Psilocybin and can potentially amplify its effects. Usually comes in confection or gum form. Helps reduces nausea especially with large doses. Sold online and at many head shops.
- *Apple cider vinegar*: May increase the bioavailability of Psilocybin and support digestion. Known to reduce nausea. Recommend taking one shot per gram of mushrooms.

1.2.6: Anecdotal Reports and Strain Variability

Many experienced Seekers of magic mushrooms report noticeable differences in active effects between strains, which could be attributed to variations in alkaloid content[27]. These anecdotal reports often describe unique combinations of visual, emotional, and cognitive

---

27 Gartz, J., Allen, J. W., & Merlin, M. D. (2004). Ethnomycology, biochemistry, and cultivation of Psilocybe samuiensis Guzmán, Bandala, and Allen, a new psychoactive fungus from Koh Samui, Thailand. Journal of Ethnopharmacology, 43(2), 73-80.

experiences associated with specific strains. Another defining factor is the perceived intensity of the overall session. However, more controlled scientific research is needed to validate these claims and identify the underlying mechanisms responsible for any observed differences between strains and Seekers' physiological variables.

In summary, while there is currently limited scientific evidence to support the idea that the various alkaloids found in magic mushrooms have synergistic properties, anecdotal reports and the *entourage effect* hypothesis lend some credibility to this theory. The entourage effect is a theory that proposes when multiple compounds, such as cannabinoids and terpenes, are present together in cannabis or other plant-based substances, they work together synergistically to produce an overall effect that is greater than the sum of their individual effects. Essentially, the entourage effect suggests that the combination of different compounds in a plant can enhance the therapeutic benefits of each individual compound by working together to create a more comprehensive therapeutic effect. This concept is often discussed in relation to the effects of cannabis, but it can also apply to other plant-based medicines. The entourage effect is an area of ongoing research in the field of plant-based medicine.

Further research into the lesser-studied alkaloids and their potential interactions with Psilocybin and psilocin is warranted. The current legal status of magic mushrooms is an obstacle to this kind of inquiry, but with time, we hope to better understand the nuances of magic mushroom journeys and the extent to which strain variability plays a role in a Seeker's perception.

CHAPTER 2

Dosing Psilocybin Mushrooms

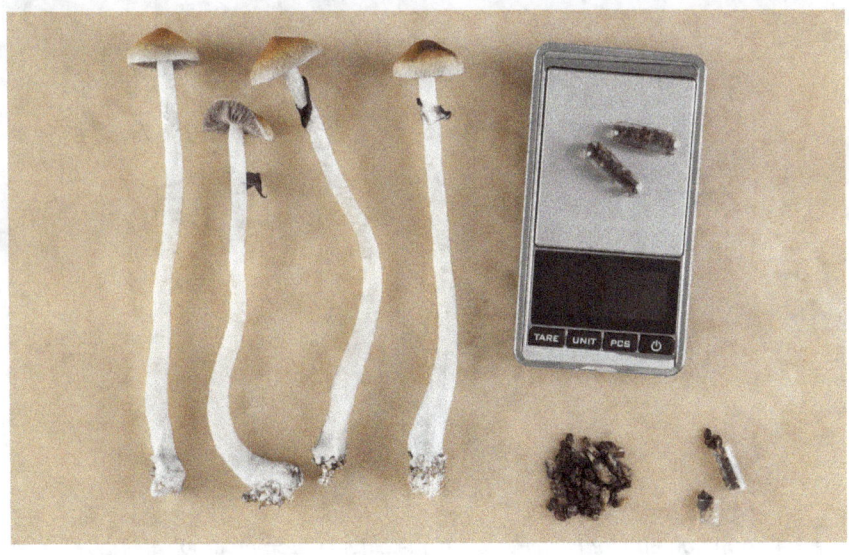

2.1 Understanding Potency

Psilocybin can only be tested for research purposes with a permit from the Drug Enforcement Administration (DEA), which prohibits public access to analytical testing services meant to ensure safety. Individuals who don't know the potency of their supply can struggle to accurately gauge the proper dosage. This can increase the risk of negative side effects or negative experiences. Since many Seekers will not have access to laboratory testing, it's important to use a scale to accurately measure the dosage and avoid consuming mushrooms based on visual estimation, which can be highly unreliable.

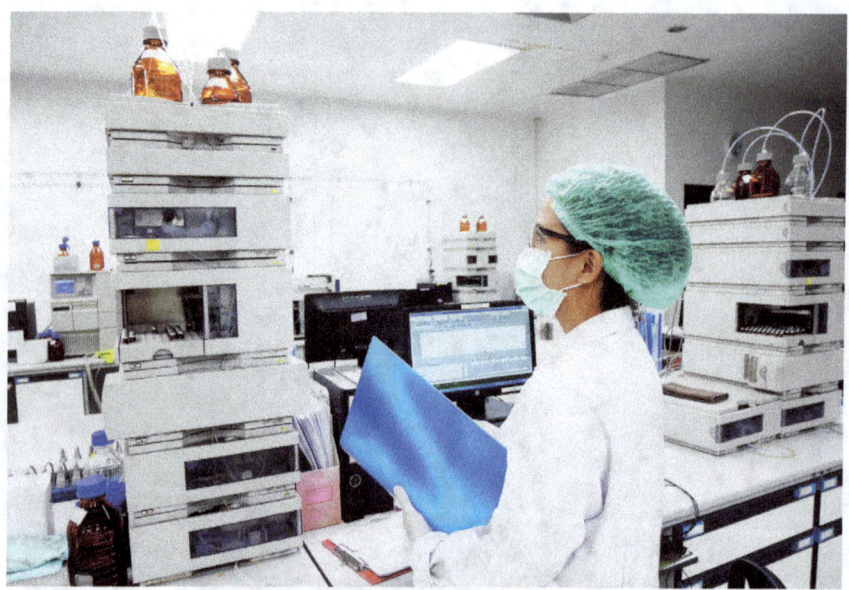

Chromatograph for High Performance Liquid Chromatography (HPLC)

2.1.1 Common Testing Methods

Scientists use a method called high-performance liquid chromatography (HPLC) to measure how strong or potent the psilocybin compound is in mushrooms. They dissolve the mushroom extract in a liquid and pass it through a tube filled with tiny particles. As the liquid moves through the tube, different compounds separate from each other based on their speed, and a detector at the end of the tube measures the separated compounds to determine their concentration levels. Using HPLC, scientists can measure the levels of psilocybin and psilocin in the mushroom samples, which helps them determine how potent or strong they are. This information can be useful for mushroom growers, researchers, and healthcare professionals who are interested in studying the effects of psilocybin. However, they require specialized equipment and expertise, making them complex to operate and inaccessible to most.

Home test kits, such as the Miraculix, provide a simpler way to estimate the psilocybin potency of mushrooms. These kits often rely on colorimetric reactions, where a chemical reagent reacts with the psychoactive compounds, resulting in a color change to the solution. The intensity of the color is proportional to the concentration of the total alkaloids, which measure Psilocybin and Psilocin. Though Psilocin does degrade more rapidly, relative to the concentration of Psilocybin, this difference is minimal. Determining potency in this way is a qualitative process, so having experience matching the shade of the reagent to the card helps. The card color is meant to be matched under sunlight or 5000K, as indoor light adds more orange tones, making the results harder to evaluate. While these tests are ±10% of HPLC's accuracy, they are more accessible and affordable for the average person.

2.1.2 Calculating Mushroom Potency

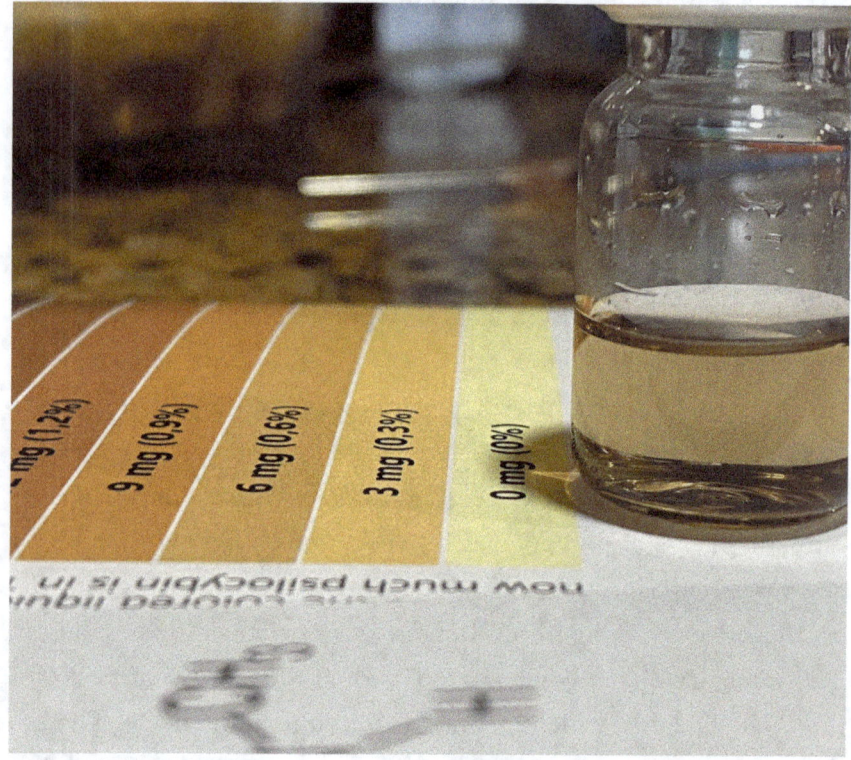

Miraculix home test kits ensure presence of potency of Psilocybin and Psilocin. This particular test-kit will measure between .3% and 2.4% total alkaloids.

Different strains of magic mushrooms can vary significantly in potency, meaning that the same weight of mushrooms from one strain may have a much stronger effect than the same amount from another strain. Psilocybin content in dried (not fresh) whole-fruit mushrooms can vary by as much as two to ten times the assumed potency.

For example, if a Golden Teacher strain of *Psilocybe Cubensis* has an *assumed* average of 1% Psilocybin potency per gram, consuming a Penis Envy at 2% means a Seeker is taking twice the assumed dose. Mushrooms in the *Psilocybe Azurescens* or *Psilocybe Cyanescens* families can be ten times the assumed potency.

Before testing was available, most people estimated their mushroom doses visually or with a scale by gross weight. In actuality, the gross weight of the mushroom fruiting bodies has very little to do with the potency of a dose. An average P. *Cubensis Tampanesis Mexicana* truffle might contain .03% psilocybin, while strains like Enigma have been tested as high as 3%. That's a range of one to one hundred times the assumed potency.

Assuming a mushroom potency of 1%, a microdose can be 50mg-200mg *cracker dry weight*, which yields 500μg-2mg Psilocybin (500μg = ~.5mg), while the average Hero trip can be 2-4g dry weight, which yields 20-40mg Psilocybin. The results vary, and the optimal dose depends on the person. Seekers should start low and slow, and keep track of their experiences to figure out dose ranges that work for their goals.

Example:

5g of dry Penis Envy at 2% potency would be calculated as:
Total psilocybin (mg) = Dry Weight (mg) * Potency (%) or
5000mg * .02 = 100mg pure psilocybin

Depending on your experience level, body weight and tolerance. 100mg is usually way too high a dose to have a productive "trip."

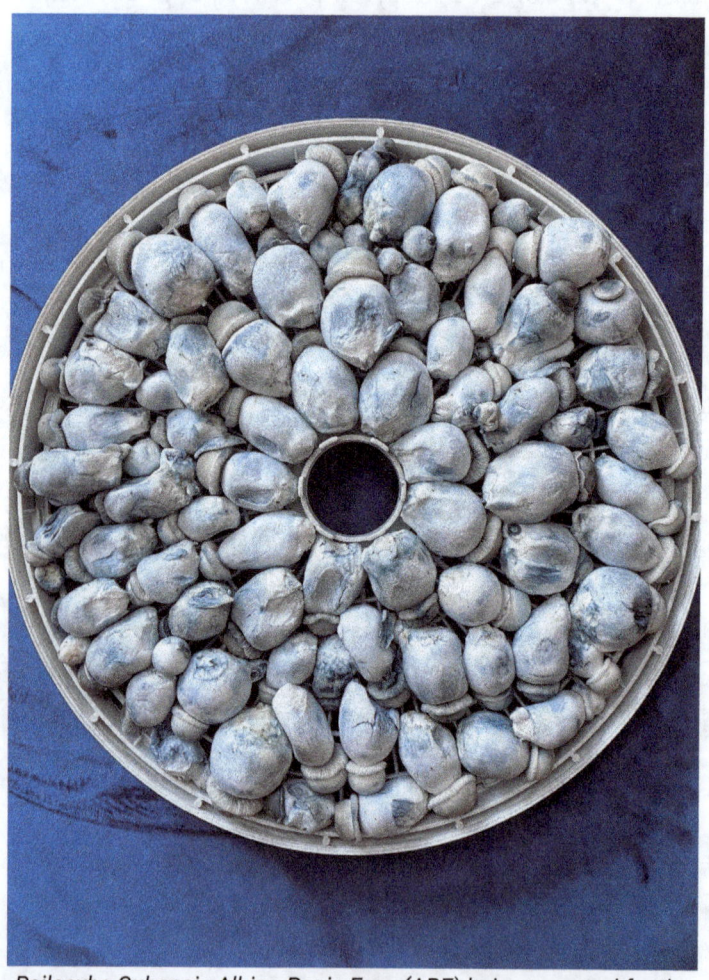

Psilocybe Cubensis Albino Penis Envy (APE) being prepared for the dehydrator.

2.3 Microdosing

Microdosing involves taking a small sub-perceptual dose of a psychedelic substance, typically around 1/10th to 1/20th of a recreational dose. This practice is intended to provide subtle benefits without inducing a full-blown 5g "Hero trip." An average microdose is 50mg-200mg and lasts for about three hours.

James Fadiman, a well-known researcher in the fields of psychedelic substances and altered states of consciousness, found one microdose per day followed by two days without microdosing psilocybin mushrooms was well-tolerated by participants and produced positive effects on mood, creativity, and focus.

Here are some tips for microdosing psilocybin mushrooms:

- It is important to start microdosing slowly and to gradually increase your dosage as needed.
- Microdosing on an empty stomach can help you feel the effects more quickly.
- The best time to microdose mushrooms can vary depending on individual preferences, daily routines, and desired outcomes. However, most people find that taking a microdose in the morning works well. This allows the effects to unfold throughout the day, providing potential benefits such as increased focus, creativity, and mood enhancement without interfering with sleep patterns at night.

- It is important to stay hydrated and listen to your body while microdosing because it knows best. People who second-guess the dose often regret it.

2.4 Dosing Cycles

One of the reasons it's essential to cycle the intake of psilocybin microdoses is to minimize the risk of developing a tolerance to the substance. Over time, your body may become accustomed to the effects of psilocybin, and this can lessen its effectiveness and negate the benefits you hoped to gain from microdosing. Cycling your intake can help avoid developing such tolerances and ensure the continuing effectiveness of the substance over time. Cycling your microdosing intake also allows you to better assess whether microdosing is beneficial to you or not. It provides you with the opportunity to take breaks and assess your situation and track your progress over time to see if there is any improvement in your mental health, creativity, or cognitive abilities.

Microdosing in cycles helps prevent the development of tolerance, ensuring the effectiveness of smaller doses[28]. Furthermore, taking breaks between microdose periods can allow the body to recover. Psilocybin may have some mild physical side effects, such as changes in appetite, sleep patterns and mood, among others. By cycling the

---

28 Fadiman, J. (2011). The Psychedelic Explorer's Guide: Safe, Therapeutic, and Sacred Journeys. Rochester, VT: Park Street Press.

microdose, you can monitor and control the extent to which you're using psilocybin to manage these side effects. There is no set duration for microdosing psilocybin mushrooms. Some people microdose for a few weeks, while others microdose for months or even years.

Are you sensitive? It is important to listen to your body and stop microdosing if you experience any negative side effects, such as nausea, headaches, gastrointestinal distress, fatigue, and sensitivity to light. Furthermore, some individuals may be more susceptible to adverse effects than others, since everyone's body may react differently to psilocybin microdoses.

Start slow and take off days in between cycles. For beginners the optimal dose depends heavily on listening to their body. On the first day begin with 50mg (.05g on a scale) and wait at least 30 minutes to see if you feel any effects. Then wait until day 5 to double the dose to 100mg (.1g) and continue increasing slowly over time to 200mg (.2g) until you feel comfortable with the amount that makes you feel best. Effects typically last 3-4 hours.

It's normal to desire a bit more later on as your system builds a tolerance to Psilocybin. An initial tolerance isn't necessarily a bad thing because you don't want it to be a negative experience. The table below shows Seekers how to progressively find their optimal microdose over a thirty day period.

Day	Dose in Grams	Phase
1	0.05	Familiarization
2	OFF	
3	OFF	
4	OFF	
5	0.1	Experimentation
6	OFF	
7	OFF	
8	OFF	
9	0.1	
10	OFF	
11	OFF	
12	0.1	
13	OFF	
14	OFF	
15	0.15	Optimization
16	OFF	
17	OFF	
18	0.15	
19	OFF	
20	OFF	
21	0.15	
22	OFF	
23	OFF	
24	0.15	
25	OFF	
26	OFF	
27	0.15	
28	OFF	
29	OFF	
30	0.2	

Dosing in cycles periodically allows time for the brain to integrate the experience and promote neuroplasticity. Cycling allows for better integration of insights or changes gained during microdosing days. Break days provide time to reflect, process, and apply information from microdosing experiences[29].

Recent research supports that you do not have to necessarily feel the psychedelic effect of the active substances to gain long-term benefits. For example, a 2020 article[30] by Olson DE in the ACS Pharmacology & Translational Science journal concludes that the long-term therapeutic benefits of psychedelics may not be dependent on the subjective effects experienced during the acute psychedelic experience. Studies have shown that even in cases where participants did not report significant acute effects, long-term benefits such as reductions in depression and anxiety symptoms were observed. This suggests that the therapeutic effects of psychedelics may involve more than just the acute subjective effects and could be related to the neural, physiological, and psychological changes induced by the compounds.

The sensation of a microdose can be compared to a gentle, warm hug. The objective is to be consistent by integrating microdosing into your daily routine as life presents its challenges. Seekers should not experience hallucinations or significant alterations in perception.

Instead, the benefits of microdosing are thought to be subtle, such as improved mood, creativity, focus, and a general sense of well-

---

29 Waldman, A. (2017). A Really Good Day: How Microdosing Made a Mega Difference in My Mood, My Marriage, and My Life. Penguin Random House.

30 https://pubs.acs.org/doi/10.1021/acsptsci.0c00192

being.[31] These benefits may not be immediately noticeable but can manifest over time as Seekers integrate microdosing into their daily lives and develop new habits or perspectives.

In our years of practice, we have found that people typically fall into two distinct dosing groups. A majority of people will be very sensitive to the effects of psilocybin and will be fine microdosing, while the rest require larger macro-doses to achieve their goals. Discovering whether you are better off microdosing or macrodosing requires some experimentation with very low doses. Slow and low microdosing is usually a great way to begin.

---

31 Anderson, T., Petranker, R., Christopher, A., Rosenbaum, D., Weissman, C., Dinh-Williams, L. A., ... & Hui, K. (2021). Psychedelic microdosing benefits and challenges: an empirical codebook. Harm Reduction Journal, 18(1), 1-17.

2.5 Macro / Hero Dosing

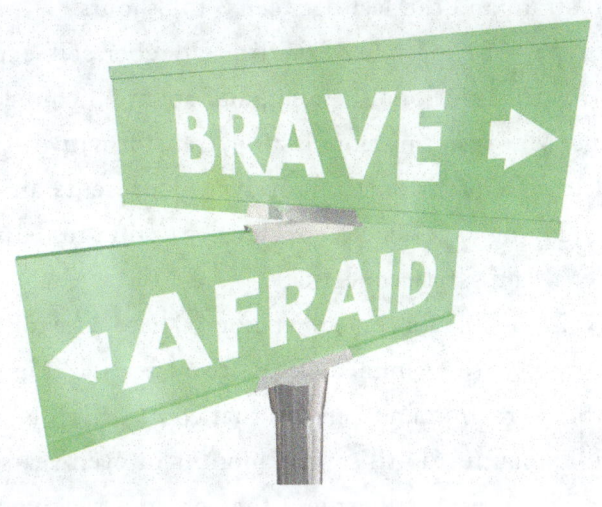

A macrodose usually refers to a high-dose of a psychedelic substance, including psilocybin, which is the active compound found in some species of magic mushrooms. A macrodose of psilocybin is typically considered to be a dose that is high enough to produce profound psychedelic effects that include changes in perception, thought, and mood. The effects of psilocybin macrodoses can last for several hours and can be accompanied by intense visual and auditory hallucinations, as well as profound insights and experiences that are often described as mystical or transformative. It is important to note that the effects of macrodosing with psilocybin can also be unpredictable and overwhelming, and should therefore only be done under the guidance of a qualified and experienced facilitator in a supportive and safe environment. A Hero dose can range from 2g - 5g depending on the person and strain and can last between 3 to 8 hours.

These types of experiences facilitate deeper self-exploration, personal growth, emotional healing, and spiritual connection in a shorter time. May result in more lasting, transformative effects after fewer and less frequent doses. However, it presents an increased risk of challenging experiences, greater disruption to daily life, and potential legal and safety concerns.

While it is possible for someone taking a "hero dose" of psilocybin mushrooms to have some immediate positive effects, it is important to note that the more profound benefits that come with this experience may not fully manifest until several months or even years after the experience. This is especially true if the person is seeking to engage in personal development work as a result of their experience. In order to fully integrate their experience and achieve the desired positive outcomes, they must be committed to doing the personal work required to gain a deeper understanding of themselves, their thoughts, and their emotions. Mindfulness is essential, not only as a regular practice, but as a mindset that can support this journey of personal development. While a "hero dose" of psilocybin mushrooms may be a powerful experience, committing to the practice and mindset of mindfulness can support continued growth and long-lasting benefits.

Individual responses to Psilocybin can vary, so start with a conservative dose and be prepared to adjust as needed. It's important to listen to your body and respect its limits. By considering your goals, intentions, and personal factors, you can make an informed decision about whether microdosing or macrodosing is right for you.

When it comes to taking heroic doses of magic mushrooms, it is important to understand that there is no universal timetable or formula that will work for everyone. The appropriate time to wait between journeys can vary depending on the individual and their own personal circumstances. However, as a general guideline, it is recommended to wait at least two to four weeks between high-dose experiences to allow for proper integration and recovery.

Recovering from a high-dose experience is an important process that allows the mind and body to fully recuperate. It can be a challenging experience as the insights and lessons gained from the journey are integrated and processed. Therefore, it is recommended to take the time to process and integrate these insights fully before embarking on another journey. In some cases, it may be beneficial to wait longer between journeys, such as several months or more, depending on one's personal growth goals and mental health.

Everyone is unique, and their experiences and insights can vary. It is essential to always listen to your body and mind, and make sure you are in a good mental and physical state before undertaking another heroic journey. Taking heroic doses of magic mushrooms can be a powerful tool for personal growth and transformation. However, it is crucial to approach this experience with respect and caution, and to create a safe and supportive environment to facilitate the journey. By respecting the process, and giving oneself ample time between journeys, one can reap the benefits and insights gained from these experiences that can positively impact their lives.

2.6 Preparing the Dose

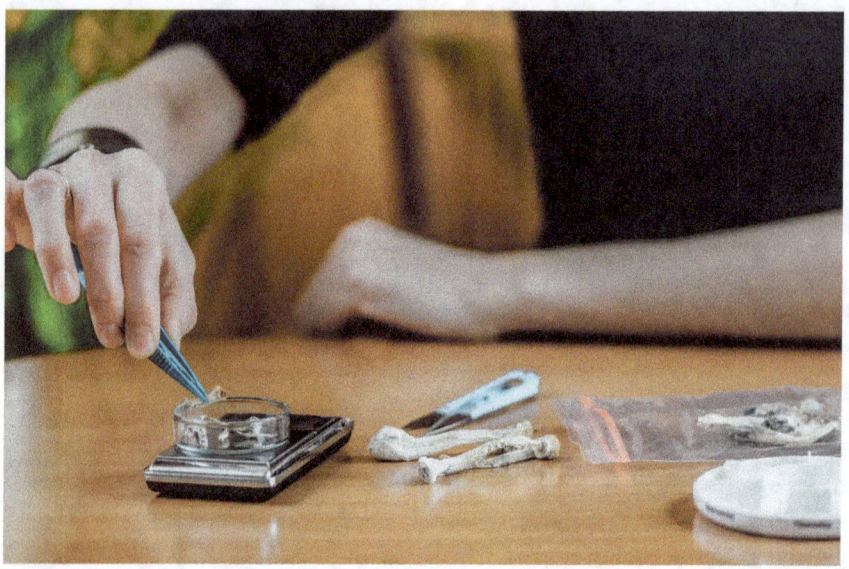

Determining the appropriate dosage for your journey is a critical component of a safe and meaningful experience. In this chapter, we will discuss microdosing to determine what's best for you. The effects of the active ingredients can vary depending on the individual, dosage, set and setting, and personal mindset. It is important to note that everyone's experience may be different.

When it comes to dried mushrooms, there are a few things to keep in mind. First, make sure the mushrooms are fully dried before consuming them. If they are still moist, they can become contaminated with bacteria or mold. Second, be aware that the potency of dried mushrooms can vary depending on how they were dried and stored.

Finally, it's important to properly measure out the dosage of dried mushrooms, as it can be more difficult to accurately determine the amount of psylocibin by weight compared to fresh mushrooms, which are usually far less potent gram for gram. However, there are several challenges that can arise when attempting to weigh mushrooms, especially if you don't have a scale.

The best type of scale to use for measuring the dosage of magic mushrooms is a digital scale that can accurately measure small amounts, such as 0.01 grams. It's important to choose a scale that has a high level of precision. Look for a scale that has a tare function, which allows

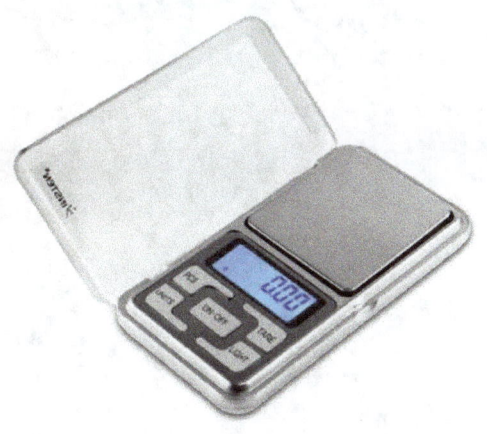

you to zero out the weight of the container you're using to hold the mushrooms. This makes it easier to get an accurate measurement of just the mushrooms. A small, portable scale that can fit in your pocket or bag is also convenient if you plan to travel with your mushrooms.

Once you know your potency, now you can use your .001 scale to measure your dose according to the following chart.

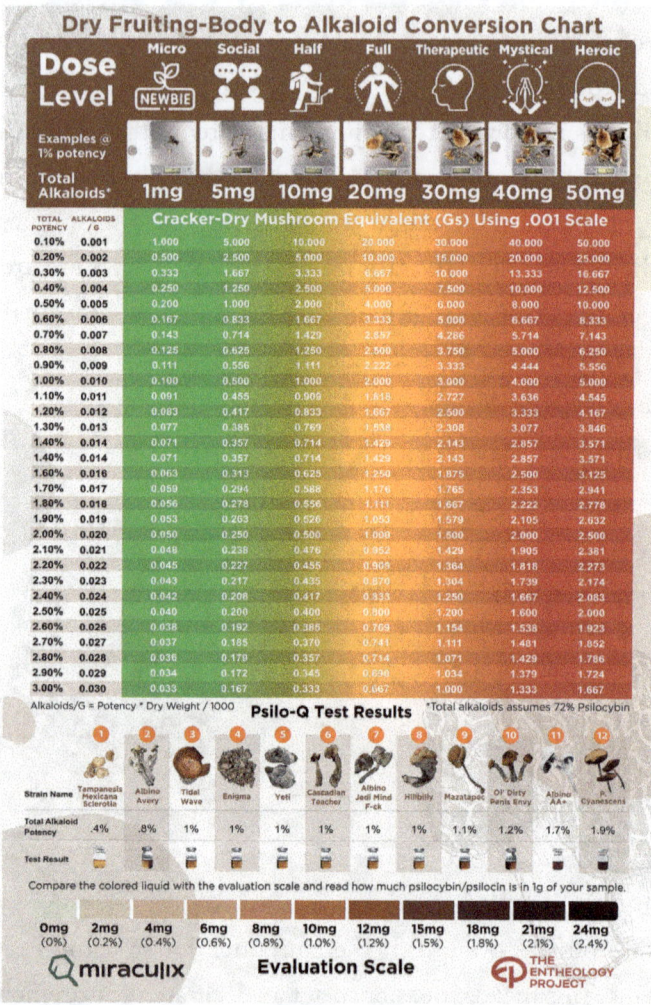

Find the dose level you'd like to achieve on the X axis and then go down to the mushroom's potency on the Y axis to find the exact dose in grams.

2.7 Took Too Much?

If you find yourself experiencing a negative psychedelic "trip," also known as a "bad trip," there are several strategies that can help you manage the situation and potentially shift it in a more positive direction.

If someone is having a challenging psychedelic trip, going to the hospital may not be the best idea, because hospitals are often not equipped to deal with psychedelic "trips." The medical staff may not have experience with psychedelic use or may not understand the nature of a psychedelic trip, which could lead to negative consequences.

Additionally, hospitals may be stressful and overwhelming environments for people in a sober frame of mind, and this impression can be exacerbated when a Seeker is under the influence of a psychedelic compound. The unfamiliar surroundings, bright lights, and medical equipment can seem frightening and disorienting, leading to additional anxiety and distress.

Furthermore, seeking medical attention could potentially result in legal or criminal consequences, as psychedelic use is not currently legal in many parts of the world. This can create a stressful situation for the individual and potentially worsen their mental state.

Instead, it's recommended that a Seeker invites a trusted friend or sitter to help navigate the experience and provide a safe and supportive environment. Techniques such as deep breathing, meditation, and changing the setting can also be helpful in calming the individual and redirecting a trip that's going in the wrong direction.

If the individual is experiencing persistent or severe distress, it's important to seek help from a mental health professional who is experienced in psychedelic therapy. The right individual can provide guidance and support in integrating the experience and addressing any underlying or pre-existing psychological issues.

If you are alone, here are some things you can do on your own:

1. Change the environment: Change the environment around you by moving to a different location or changing the lighting. This shift may help change the focus of the trip and alleviate negative feelings.
2. Practice deep breathing: Deep breathing can help promote a sense of calm and relaxation and provide oxygen to the brain, which can help reduce feelings of anxiety.
3. Practice meditation: Meditation can help calm the mind and redirect thoughts. There are specific meditation techniques, such as mindfulness, that are designed to help during a difficult "trip."
4. Engage with a trusted friend: Sometimes just talking to someone during a difficult or challenging trip can help alleviate negative feelings. It's important to have a trusted friend who can assist, reassure and support during a difficult "trip."
5. Listen to music: Listening to calming music can help relax and distract the mind from negative thoughts.
6. Consume something sweet: Some people find that eating something sweet, like candy or chocolate, can help reduce feelings of anxiety and provide a quick burst of energy.

7. Remember that the experience will end: Remembering that the effects of psilocybin are temporary and that the experience will end can alleviate anxiety and help one stay focused on the present moment.

8. Practice breathwork: Breathwork can be an effective tool to help calm someone experiencing an intense or overwhelming dose of magic mushrooms. It works by helping the individual regain a sense of control, grounding them in the present moment, and regulating their nervous system.

Here are some ways breathwork can assist during a challenging psychedelic experience:

-   Activating the parasympathetic nervous system: Controlled and mindful breathing activates the parasympathetic nervous system, which is responsible for the "rest and digest" response. This counteracts the "fight or flight" response triggered by the sympathetic nervous system during moments of stress or anxiety. As a result, the individual practicing breathwork experiences a reduction in heart rate, blood pressure, and overall anxiety levels.

-   Grounding in the present moment: Focusing on the breath can bring the individual's awareness back to the present awareness, helping them to feel more grounded and connected to their body in time and space. This can be particularly helpful during a psychedelic experience, where one's perception of reality may be altered.

- Regaining a sense of control: By taking control of their breath, the individual can regain a sense of peace over their experience. This can help to reduce feelings of panic or helplessness that may arise during a challenging "trip."
- Reducing hyperventilation: Rapid or shallow breathing can exacerbate feelings of anxiety and panic. By consciously slowing and deepening the breath, the Seeker can counteract the physiological effects of hyperventilation, leading to a calmer state.

Remember that each person's experience is unique, and what works for you might not be effective for someone else. It is essential to remain calm, patient, and compassionate toward yourself, and adapt your approach to your specific needs and circumstances. Note that these can vary from experience to experience, so you'll want to make arrangements for relaxation ahead of time, if possible. By practicing these strategies, you can better navigate challenging moments during a psychedelic experience and potentially shift your perspective toward a more positive and meaningful journey.

CHAPTER 3

Psilocybin

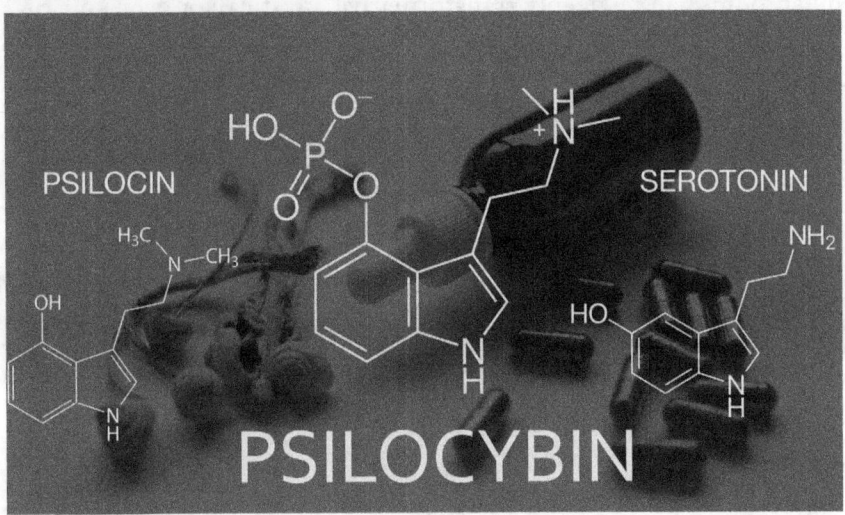

3.1 Psilocybin the "Magic" Alkaloid

Magic mushrooms contain the active alkaloid Psilocybin, a naturally occurring psychedelic molecule found in over two hundred species of mushrooms. Psilocybin is the fungi's defensive compound, whose original purpose was to teach hungry beings a valuable lesson if they dared to consume the mushroom carrying this chemical.

However, some early humans were not deterred, and at some point, started to ingest these active strains of mushrooms intentionally. The reason for this is related to why the mushrooms are called "magic": they have the ability to induce profound changes in perception, emotion, and consciousness. The experiences brought on by magic mushrooms can be deeply transformative, mystical, or even spiritual for some individuals, giving these fungi a seemingly magical quality.

Mushrooms containing psilocybin have been used for centuries by indigenous cultures for spiritual and therapeutic purposes, and, more recently, they have gained attention for their active ingredients' potential in treating various mental health conditions, such as depression, anxiety, and PTSD.

When psilocybin-containing mushrooms are ingested, the psilocybin is rapidly converted into its active form, *psilocin*, within the body. This conversion occurs primarily in the liver, where the enzyme alkaline phosphatase removes a phosphate group from psilocybin, transforming it into psilocin (a process known as "de-phosphorylation"). However, this conversion can also take place to a lesser extent in the gut as well, since the same enzyme is present throughout the digestive tract.

Psilocin primarily acts on the brain by binding to and activating specific serotonin receptors, most notably the 5-HT2A. This receptor subtype is widely distributed throughout the brain and plays a significant role in modulating perception, cognition, and mood. Serotonin is a crucial neurotransmitter involved in regulating mood, memory, appetite, and sleep, among other functions.

PSILOCIN   SEROTONIN

The molecular structure of psilocin is very similar to that of serotonin, meaning Psilocin easily binds to the 5-HT2A receptor.

The gut also contains serotonin receptors, as serotonin plays a crucial role in regulating various gastrointestinal functions, such as motility, secretion, and sensation. In fact, it is estimated that around 95% of the body's total serotonin is found in the gut.[32] During the titration process, the body absorbs the converted psilocin from the gut and bloodstream, transporting it across the blood-brain barrier to reach the central nervous system.

This activation leads to a cascade of neural signaling, which produces the altered states of perception, cognition, and emotion that are characteristic of a psychedelic experience. As the body gradually metabolizes psilocin and clears it from the system via the liver, the intensity of the effects diminishes, bringing the individual back to their normal state of consciousness.

---

32 Mawe, G.M., & Hoffman, J.M., "Serotonin signaling in the gut--functions, dysfunctions and therapeutic targets," Nature Reviews Gastroenterology & Hepatology, 2013, https://www.nature.com/articles/nrgastro.2013.105.

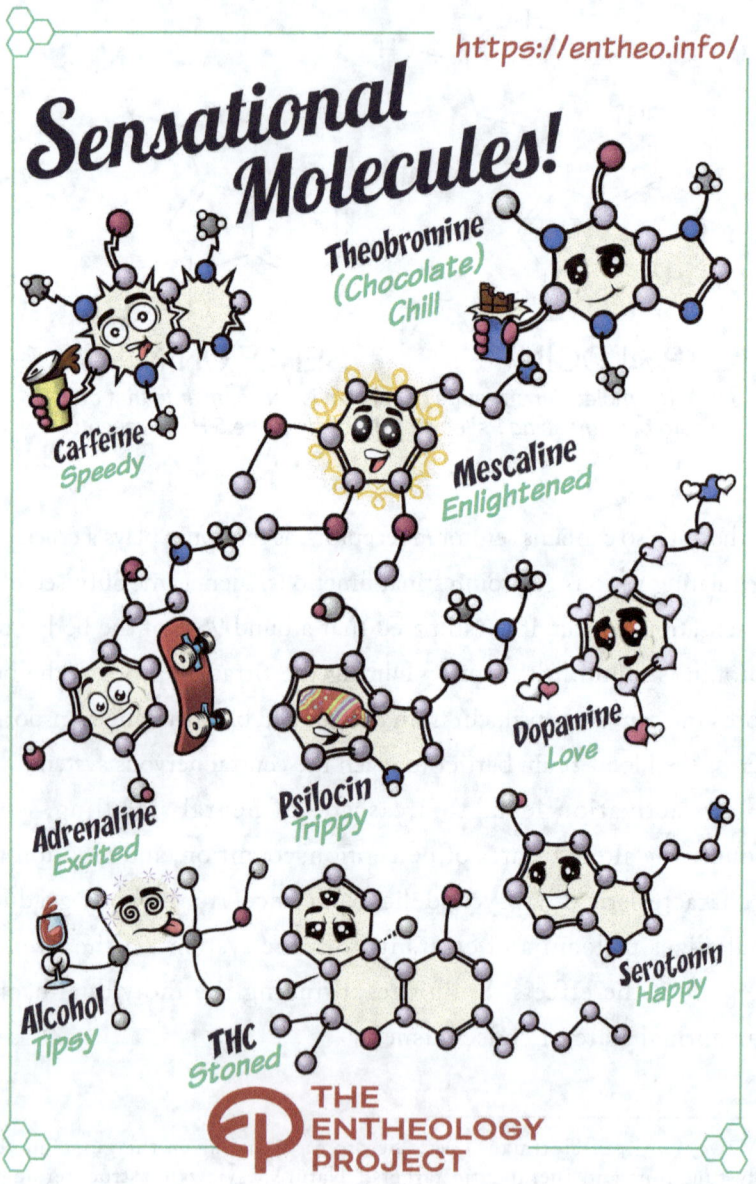

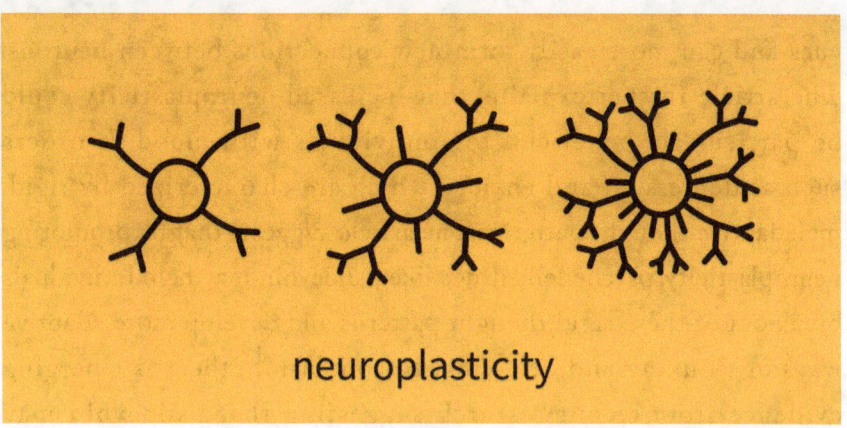

neuroplasticity

Enhanced neuroplasticity: One source that supports the statement that psilocybin may promote neuroplasticity is a review article titled "The Neurobiology of Psychedelic Drugs: Implications for the Treatment of Mood Disorders" published in the journal Nature Reviews Neuroscience (Carhart-Harris and Nutt, 2017). This article summarizes recent research on the effects of psychedelic drugs on the brain and highlights the potential therapeutic benefits of these drugs, including their ability to promote neuroplasticity. The article explains that recent studies using brain imaging techniques such as functional magnetic resonance imaging (fMRI) and magnetoencephalography (MEG) have shown that psilocybin can increase functional connectivity between different regions of the brain, particularly the default mode network (DMN), which is known to be involved in self-referential thinking and rumination. The article suggests that this increased connectivity may reflect a state of heightened neuroplasticity, where the brain is more responsive to environmental cues and can more easily form new connections between neurons. The article further explains that increased neuroplasticity could be particularly beneficial for individuals with mood disorders such as depression and anxiety, which are characterized by rigid, maladaptive thought patterns. The article suggests that by promoting neuroplasticity, psychedelic drugs like psilocybin may help individuals break out of these rigid thought patterns and develop more adaptive ways of thinking and behaving. In conclusion, there is emerging evidence from recent research suggesting that psilocybin may promote neuroplasticity in the brain. This effect could be particularly beneficial for individuals suffering from mental health conditions characterized by rigid, maladaptive thought patterns.

The capacity for the brain to adapt and change through neuroplasticity can vary throughout a person's life, but generally, it appears to slow down as we age. The bulk of neuroplastic changes are observed during early childhood and adolescence, and research suggests that the brain becomes less adaptable as we move towards adulthood and beyond. While adult brains are still undergoing neuroplastic changes, these changes tend to be less profound and occur more slowly than in younger brains. Despite this, it is important to note that the brain remains adaptable throughout life, and it is never too late to learn new things or work on improving cognitive and emotional function. Engaging in activities that challenge the mind, such as learning a new language or a musical instrument, can help to stimulate neuronal activity and promote neuroplasticity. Regular exercise and mindfulness practices may also be beneficial in promoting neuroplasticity and maintaining cognitive function throughout life.

- *BDNF upregulation*: Brain-derived neurotrophic factor (BDNF) is a protein that plays a crucial role in the growth, survival, and maintenance of neurons. Research has suggested that psychedelic compounds, including Psilocybin, may increase the expression of BDNF, which could promote neurogenesis, especially later in life, and support overall brain health[33].

- *Potential neuroprotective effects*: Although direct evidence for Psilocin's neuroprotective effects is limited because of the scarcity of robust human studies, its influence on BDNF expression as well as its anti-inflammatory properties, may contribute to its potential neuroprotective effects[34].

- *Promotion of Neurogenesis*: Magic mushrooms are believed to promote *neurogenesis* (the generation of new neurons). While it is true that adult neurogenesis was once thought to be absent or very limited in the adult brain, recent research has shown that neurogenesis can indeed occur in certain regions of the adult brain. Psilocybin has been shown to promote neurogenesis in rodents, although research on this topic is still in its early stages and more research is needed to determine if this effect is also seen in humans. It is worth noting that while the brain has a limited capacity

---

33 Catlow, B. J., Song, S., Paredes, D. A., Kirstein, C. L., & Sanchez-Ramos, J. (2013). Effects of Psilocybin on hippocampal neurogenesis and extinction of trace fear conditioning. Experimental Brain Research, 228(4), 481-491.

34 Catlow, B. J., Song, S., Paredes, D. A., Kirstein, C. L., & Sanchez-Ramos, J. (2013). Effects of Psilocybin on hippocampal neurogenesis and extinction of trace fear conditioning. Experimental Brain Research, 228(4), 481-491.

for neurogenesis in certain regions, this does not mean that we stop producing neurons altogether. In fact, neurogenesis occurs throughout the lifespan to some extent, although the rate and extent of neurogenesis may decline as we age. Additionally, research has shown that there are several lifestyle factors that can support neurogenesis and overall brain health, such as regular physical exercise and a healthy diet.

- *Emotional amplification*: Psilocybin can heighten emotional experiences, making Seekers more receptive to positive emotions such as love, joy, and empathy. This emotional amplification can help individuals confront and process difficult emotions, leading to lasting therapeutic benefits.

While psilocybin has the potential to amplify positive emotions, it can also amplify negative emotions and lead to difficult experiences, known as "bad" "trips." In some cases, these negative experiences can be harmful and lead to adverse effects on mental health. It should be noted that the experience of using psilocybin is highly variable and dependent on several factors, including the person's mindset, setting, and dosage. Therefore, psilocybin should only be used under a controlled setting with a trained guide or therapist to minimize the risk of negative experiences and to ensure that the experience is therapeutic and beneficial.

3.2 The Psychedelic "Trip"

The physical effects of magic mushrooms varies from person to person and depends on factors such as the dosage, individual sensitivity, and the specific strain of mushroom used.

The effects of psilocybin ingestion vary depending on the dose and individual factors, but they can include altered perception of time, space, and self, enhanced emotions, and spiritual or mystical experiences. Some people report feeling a heightened sense of visual and auditory perception, intensified or unusual emotional states, and a greater connection to nature or their own spirituality, while others may experience confusion, anxiety, or paranoia. This why it's best to start low and slow.

Many Seekers describe a pleasant body high, or a feeling of warmth and tingling throughout their body. This sensation may be accompanied by a sense of relaxation and well-being.

Some people experience mild to moderate to excruciating nausea during the onset, which usually subsides as the experience progresses. Eating the mushrooms on an empty stomach or consuming them with ginger or lemon may help to alleviate this symptom.

Exploring the effects of magic mushrooms requires considering both the mindset of the individual and the environment in which they are consumed. These two factors are often referred to as "set" and "setting," respectively. An individual's mindset, which is shaped by their expectations and intentions for the experience, can influence the psychological effects of the mushrooms, such as changes in mood and thought patterns. Meanwhile, the physical space in which the mushrooms are consumed -- the setting -- can also greatly affect the overall experience. Consuming mushrooms in a relaxed, comfortable environment surrounded by supportive friends, for example, is likely to result in a more positive experience than consuming them in a stressful, unfamiliar setting. Taken together, set and setting are key factors that significantly influence the outcomes of a psilocybin experience and should be carefully considered in order to elicit a positive, meaningful outcome.

3.2.1 Common Positive Effects

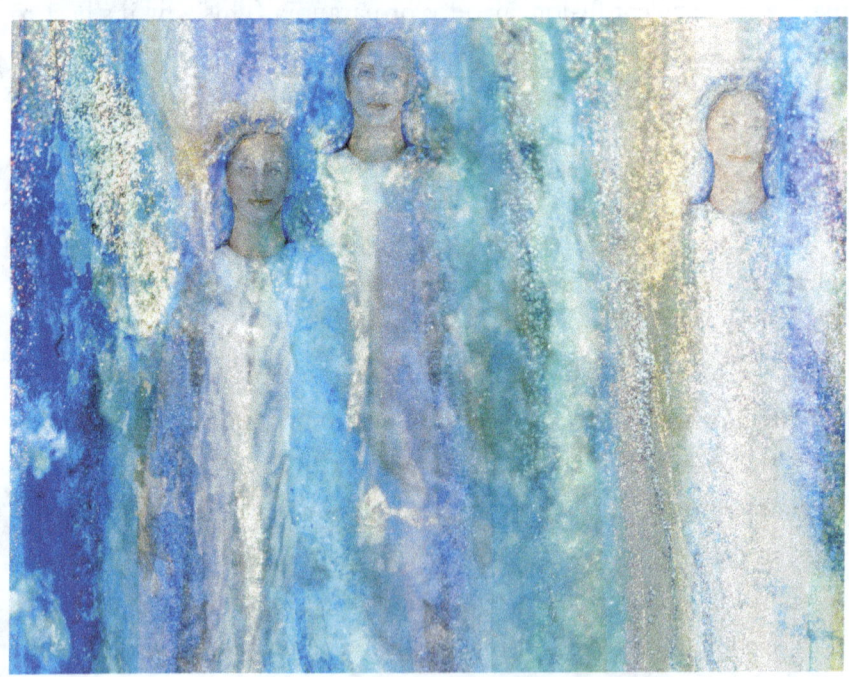

The "golden hangover" is a term used to describe a feeling of positivity and well-being that some people experience the day after taking psilocybin mushrooms. The reason behind this phenomena is not fully understood, but some researchers believe that it may be due to the way that psilocybin interacts with the brain.

According to a study published in ACS Chemical Neuroscience in 2018, researchers found that participants who took psilocybin reported increased ratings of positive moods and social effects the day after taking the drug. They also found that this effect appeared to be tied to the intensity of the participant's mystical experiences while under the influence of psilocybin. Moreover, a study published in the Journal of Psychopharmacology in 2016, found similar results in which participants reported increased positive moods and attitudes, as well as a decrease in distress and anxiety, in the days and weeks following psilocybin use. These studies suggest that the "golden hangover" is a real phenomenon that appears to be related to psilocybin use, but further research is necessary to fully understand the mechanisms behind it.

During a psilocybin experience, Seekers may have a range of intense emotional experiences, including feelings of happiness, awe, and connection to others and the world around them. These experiences can have a lasting impact on mood and outlook, leading to feelings of positivity and well-being for a period of time.

However, it's important to note that the effects of psilocybin can be highly variable and depend on a range of factors, including the dosage, setting, and individual differences in brain chemistry, physiology, and psychology. Others may have a different experience, such as feeling tired or emotionally drained.

It's also worth noting that the long-term effects of psilocybin on mood and well-being are still being studied, and more research is needed to fully understand the potential benefits and risks of using psilocybin for mental health purposes.

Here are some experiences that might occur during this period:

- *Enhanced mood*: Feelings of euphoria, joy, and emotional well-being are commonly reported.
- *Increased creativity*: Many Seekers experience heightened imagination, creativity, and a greater appreciation for art and music.
- *Deep introspection*: Psilocybin mushrooms can facilitate profound impact, enabling individuals to explore their thoughts, emotions, and beliefs.
- *Spiritual experiences*: Some Seekers report feelings of interconnectedness, unity, and a sense of the divine or transcendent.
- *Personal growth*: Many people find that their experiences with Psilocybin mushrooms lead to lasting positive changes in their lives, including increased self-awareness, empathy, and a greater sense of purpose.
- *Enhanced sensory perception*: Colors may appear more vivid, sounds may be more intense, and tactile sensations may be heightened.

3.2.2 Possible Undesired Effects

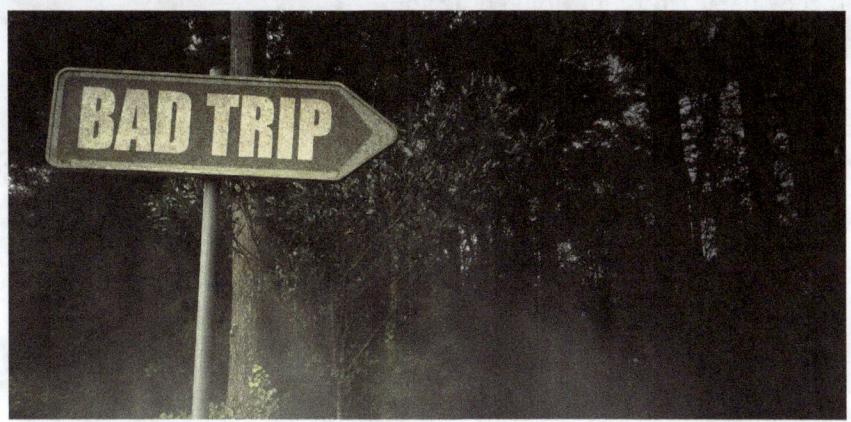

There's no such thing as a "bad" trip - just one you're not prepared for! While the use of psilocybin can have positive effects, it also has the potential to elicit a range of unwanted, subjective effects. These may include fear, anxiety, paranoia, confusion, and agitation, which typically occur during the acute phase. In rare cases, use of psilocybin can also induce psychotic episodes and long-term changes in personality, although such occurrences are extremely rare. One of the most significant risks associated with psilocybin use is the potential for a "bad trip" which can be a highly distressing and uncomfortable experience. This can involve feelings of extreme fear, anxiety, or panic, and it may be exacerbated by the individual's pre-existing mental health conditions. Furthermore, psilocybin use can lead to physical effects including nausea, vomiting, and diarrhea, which are often experienced during the onset of the effects. These side effects can be very distressing and uncomfortable, particularly if they persist for a prolonged period.

A "bad trip" is a common phrase used to describe the experience of psilocybin Seekers when they undergo a negative, fearful, and uncomfortable experience. A "bad," or difficult trip, can evoke intense negative emotions such as anxiety, paranoia, and panic, which could be overwhelming and lead to a traumatic experience. In some cases, Seekers may experience visual or auditory hallucinations that seem real and can increase feelings of distress or disorientation. It's important to note that not everyone experiences a bad trip, and some people report only positive effects from psilocybin use. Still, it's hard to predict how an individual will respond to psilocybin, and the outcome would depend on multiple factors, including the Seeker's mood, environment, and dose of the drug. Furthermore, research shows that an individual's set and setting can greatly influence the onset and experience of a "trip." Therefore, it is advisable that if one decides to take psilocybin, they should take it under the guidance of a trained and experienced therapist or in a safe, supportive, and comfortable environment. This way, the risks associated with a psilocybin trip could be mitigated, and one can feel more comfortable and positive, and therefore improve the overall experience.

In addition to the possible negative effects during acute intoxication, there is also some evidence to suggest that repeated use of psilocybin could lead to potential long-term risks. For example, an individual may develop changes in their mood or personality traits, such as increased neuroticism, decreased openness, and increased introversion. However, it is important to note that more research is required to investigate these potential risks.

Common symptoms of a difficult trip:

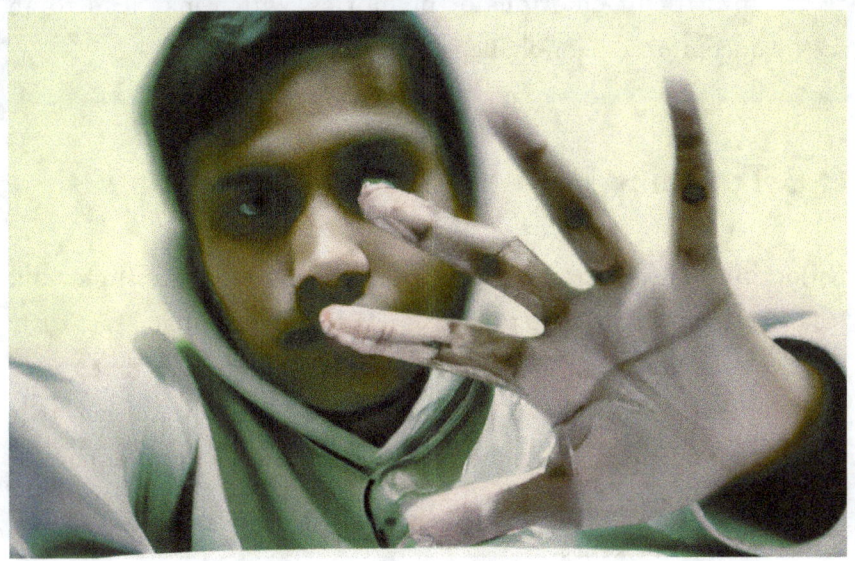

- *Hallucinations*: While many Seekers find the visual and auditory hallucinations that come with psilocybin use to be enjoyable, these experiences can be distressing for others, especially if they are not prepared for these effects.
- *Anxiety*: Some Seekers may experience heightened anxiety or paranoia, especially if they are predisposed to these feelings or if the set and setting are not conducive to a positive experience.
- *Nausea*: Ingesting Psilocybin mushrooms can cause stomach discomfort and nausea in some individuals.
- *Confusion*: Some Seekers may experience disorientation, confusion, or difficulty focusing during their "trip."

- *Challenging emotions*: Psilocybin mushrooms can bring up difficult emotions or memories, which may lead to an uncomfortable or challenging experience.

3.3 Toxicity Levels

Psilocybin mushrooms have a relatively low toxicity threshold, and it is just about impossible to consume a lethal dose. The exact toxic dose for humans is not well-established, as there have been very few confirmed cases of fatal psilocybin mushroom poisoning. It is essential to note that individual reactions can vary, and other factors, such as pre-existing health conditions or drug interactions, can influence the outcomes.

A study published in 1984 estimated the median lethal dose (LD50) of psilocybin for rats to be 280 milligrams per kilogram of body weight. However, this may not accurately translate to humans. Assuming a rough conversion, some sources suggest that a person would have to consume tens or even hundreds of grams of dried psilocybin mushrooms to potentially reach toxic levels, which is much higher than the standard recreational dose of around 1-5 grams.

3.4 Recreational Use

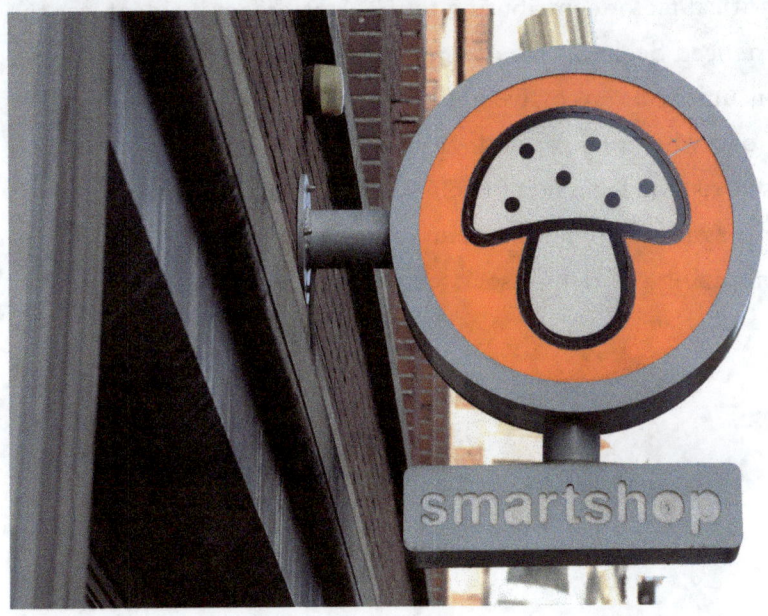

In 2008, some incidents[35] occurred in Amsterdam where tourists who had consumed hallucinogenic mushrooms engaged in dangerous and harmful behaviors, including self-harm and accidental deaths. While it's uncertain if other substances were mixed with the mushrooms, it's clear that the individuals' impaired judgment and altered perceptions played a role in their behavior. As a result of these events, the Dutch government responded by implementing stricter regulations on the sale and possession of hallucinogenic mushrooms. The new rules

---

35 https://www.dutchnews.nl/news/2008/08/teenager_dies_in_magic_mushroo/

placed an emphasis on the need for education and responsible use to minimize the risks associated with consuming these substances.

A critical factor contributing to the Amsterdam incident was the inexperienced Seekers' lack of knowledge about appropriate dosing.

Consuming an excessive amount of psilocybin mushrooms can lead to overwhelming psychological effects, impaired judgment, and increased risk of accidents or self-harm. Understanding the correct dosage for one's individual tolerance and experience level is crucial for minimizing the risks associated with psilocybin use.

CHAPTER 4

Forms of Magic Mushrooms

When looking to source Psilocybin mushrooms, it's crucial that interested Seekers prioritize safety and reliability to ensure a positive and secure experience. Always keep in mind that every individual reacts differently to various forms of mushrooms, so it's important to experiment and start slow. In this chapter, we will discuss various ways to obtain mushrooms and how to navigate safety concerns, as well as explore more dependable sources like religious organizations, psychedelic societies, and mushroom retreats.

4.1 Whole-Fruiting Bodies

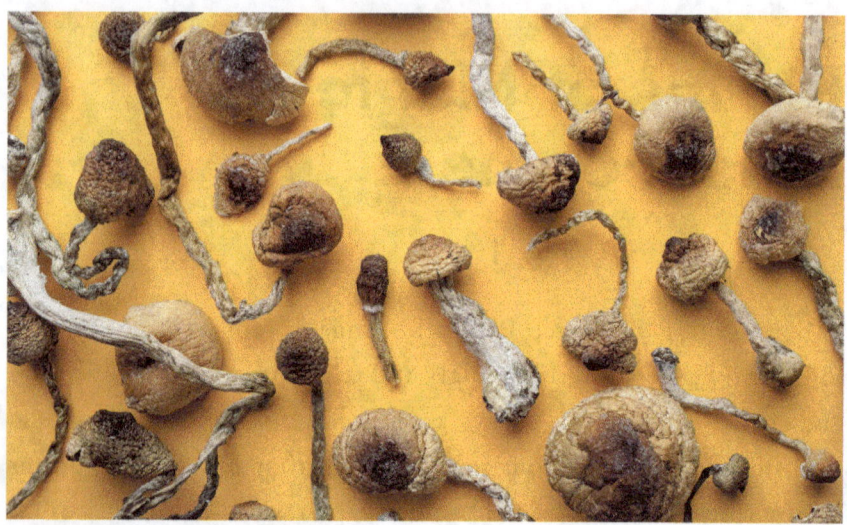

As the world of psychedelic edibles continues to evolve, enthusiasts are often faced with many options for psilocybin consumption. The main choice is between consuming the dried fruiting bodies of mushrooms, or their extracted counterparts. This section delves into the pros and cons of each option, helping you make an informed choice.

Harvesting wild Psilocybin mushrooms or cultivating them at home can both be options for procuring active strains. However, foraging is only for advanced Seekers with prior experience. It is crucial to have extensive knowledge about mushroom identification, as many toxic look-alikes can pose serious health risks if consumed. Potency varies wildly from one strain to another.

Without proper testing, 1g of a particular strain could give you a HUGE trip you may not be ready for! Ensure you are familiar with local laws regarding mushroom collection and cultivation.

Raw or dried mushrooms can be eaten directly, but they have a strong and often unpleasant taste. Mixing them with food or drink can help make the experience more enjoyable.

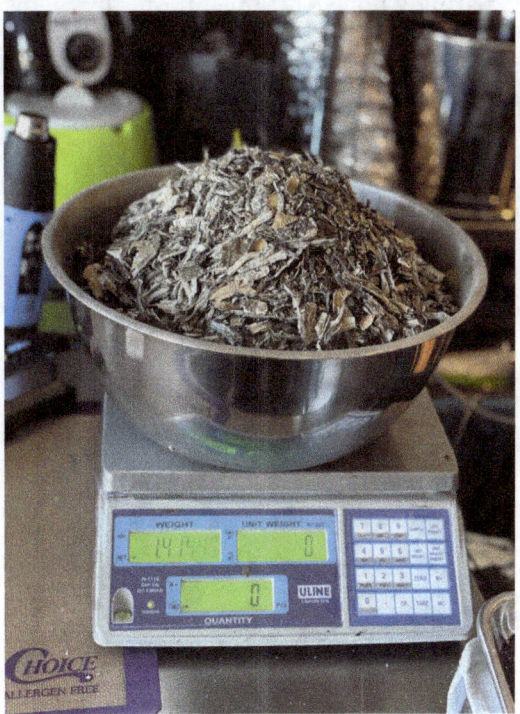

P.Cubensis Hillbilly before pulverizing.

The use of whole-fruit mushrooms in the form of edibles offers certain advantages:

1. *Natural composition*: The untouched form of whole-fruit mushrooms provides a more holistic experience due to the presence of additional compounds that may interact synergistically.
2. *Simplicity*: Incorporating whole-fruit mushrooms in recipes is relatively simple and straightforward, as it does not require additional extraction processes.
3. *Lower cost*: Eating whole-fruit mushrooms by themselves or using them in recipes can be more budget-friendly, as the extraction process can be costly and labor-intensive.

However, there are some drawbacks to using whole-fruit mushrooms:

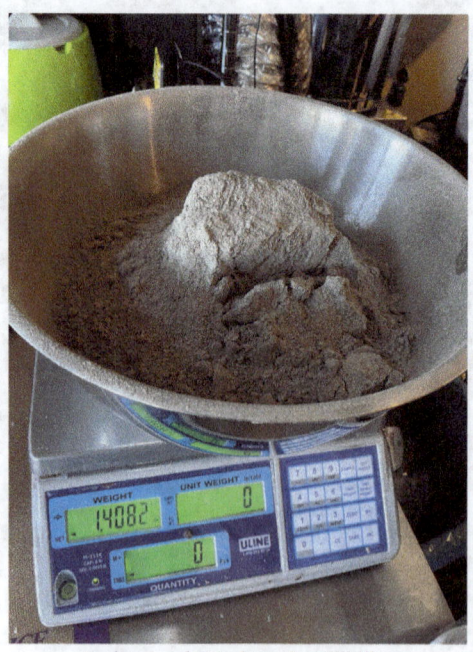

Pulverized P.Cubensis Hillbilly.

1. *Inconsistent potency*: Levels of psychoactive compounds can vary between strains and even individual flushes, making it difficult to determine an accurate dosage.
2. *Taste and texture*: Some people find the taste and texture of whole-fruit mushrooms unpalatable, affecting the overall enjoyment of the either the mushroom by itself or the edible created with it.
3. *Digestive issues*: Whole-fruit mushrooms contain fibrous chitin in their cell walls, which may cause digestive discomfort or other side effects for some individuals.

4.2 Extracts

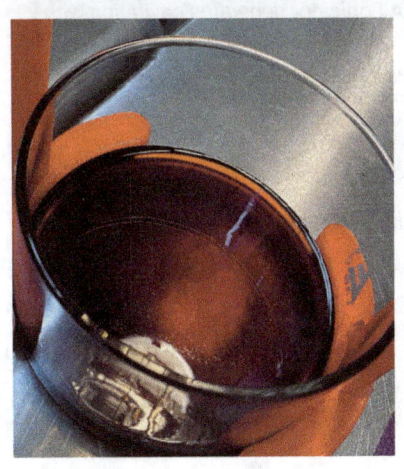

Another option for magic mushroom consumption is the creation of psilocybin extract, which can then be used in several ways. When consuming concentrated mushrooms, however, a safety concern can arise in the form of accumulated contamination by heavy metals such as lead, cadmium, and mercury and other toxins.[36]

---

36 Johnson, M. W., Garcia-Romeu, A., & Griffiths, R. R. (2017). Long-term follow-up of psilocybin-facilitated smoking cessation. The American Journal of Drug and Alcohol Abuse, 43(1), 55–60. doi: 10.1080/00952990.2016.1170135.

This is because mushrooms are very efficient at absorbing and accumulating these substances from the environment in which they are grown, and if the mushrooms' desirable compounds are concentrated, so are the undesirable ones. Concentration levels of heavy metals and other toxins in mushrooms can vary greatly depending on the substrates in which they are grown and the competency of the grower.

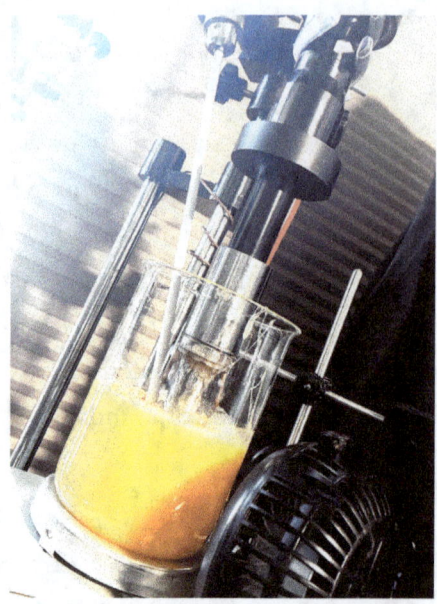

A Sonicator generates cavitation with ultrasonic frequency to create tiny bubbles that strip the soluble compounds from the mushroom fibers into a pure ethanol or methanol solution.

Extracts are usually made in a lab and are then used to make edible gummies, because trying to make gummies with whole-fruit tends to make them sludgy and green. Extracts are very difficult to make and handle property, and aspiring home extractors are advised to never try this process without a proper fume hood. There are also upsides to the extraction method. Seekers report almost no GI issues as these extracts digest quickly, and onset time is reduced.

Extracted mushrooms provide their own unique set of advantages:

1. *Consistent potency*: Extracted mushrooms offer a more controlled and consistent level of psychoactive compounds, allowing for more accurate dosing.

2. *Improved taste and texture*: The incorporation of extracts into edibles does not alter their taste and texture as significantly as whole-fruit mushrooms, potentially leading to a more enjoyable experience.

3. Reduced side effects: Extracts typically do not contain fibrous chitin, and this may reduce the likelihood of digestive issues.

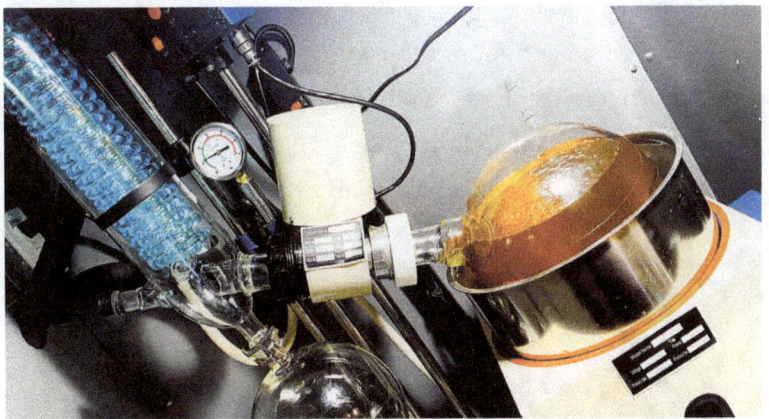

Reduction must be done in a Rotary Evaporator to reduce the liquid solution to a more concentrated extract.

However, there are disadvantages to using extracted mushrooms:

1. *Potential contaminants:* Sonicators used for extraction can leach titanium into the solution and poorly managed substrates can leach toxins into the mushrooms, which can then be concentrated to dangerous levels.

2. *Loss of synergistic effects:* The extraction process may remove or alter some compounds that contribute to the overall experience,

potentially diminishing the entourage effect – the perceived change in experiences brought on by the differing combinations of alkaloids and triterpenes in each strain.

3. *Cost and complexity*: Extracting mushrooms is labor-intensive and may require specialized equipment, increasing costs and complicating the process. Poor extraction yields also raise the final product price.

4. *Poor yields*: The active ingredients in magic mushrooms are very hard to extract, so the process often results in a 40-60% loss of the mushrooms' original weight, which dramatically raises how much raw material you need to buy in order to achieve enough extract.

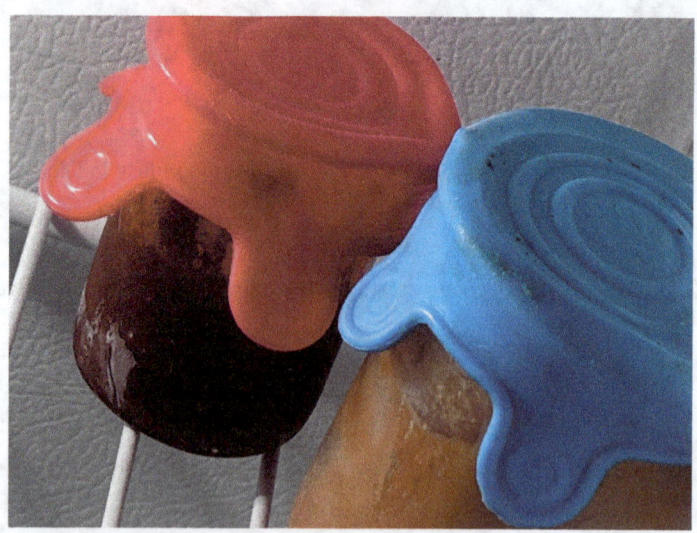

Once the mushroom Chitin fibers are filtered off and reduced, what is left is a highly bio-available magic resin. Albino strains have less color, so they extract in an orange shade (right).

4.3 Edibles

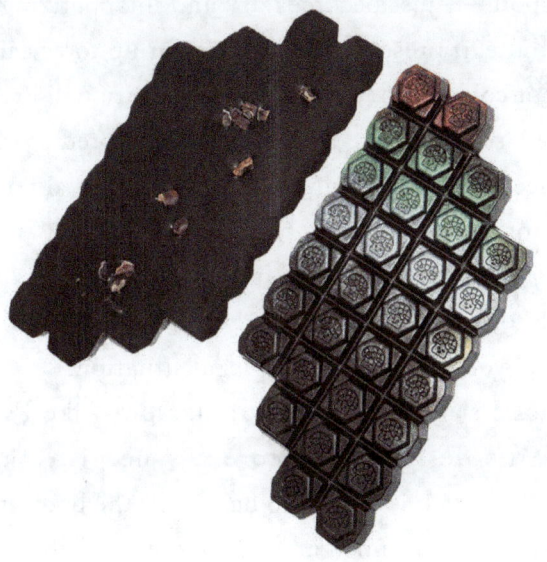

As the legal landscape surrounding psychedelic substances continues to shift, the market for mushroom edibles has experienced unprecedented growth. This trend has been driven by several factors, including increased public interest, emerging scientific research, and changing social attitudes. In this chapter, we explore the key drivers of the mushroom edible market's expansion, along with the challenges and opportunities it presents.

Psilocybin edibles are manufactured in various forms, offering different methods of consumption to cater to individual preferences. Some of the most common forms of Psilocybin edibles include:

Magic chocolates: Mushroom chocolate can be quite intense in higher doses, so please don't underestimate it! Chocolate really doesn't spoil—it just becomes dry and unappetizing. Due to this attribute, it preserves Psilocybin for up to a year, as long as it's kept cold and dry. Light and moisture will break down Psilocybin, so make sure the chocolate is stored correctly. An ideal place for safekeeping is an airtight container inside a refrigerator drawer. Though be careful, especially with magic edibles that look delicious, as chocolate bars can attract minors. Should a child unwittingly consume your edibles, you might find yourself in a serious legal situation.

Cacao is a natural carrier of alkaloids like Psilocybin because it's designed to store a synergistic alkaloid, *Theobromine* which is known to help relax the body and mind. Chocolate can help mitigate G.I. issues and the sugar can heighten a psychedelic experience.

Properly designed bars by reputable companies will offer small portions for more precise dosage control. Edibles from these companies will also have been created with good homogenization methods, which will ensure even infusion of the mushroom fruiting bodies.

Psilocybin mushroom-infused chocolates often use whole fruit to keep costs low. However, the dosage and quality of these products can vary, making it difficult to gauge their potency from one serving to the next. Exercise caution when consuming edibles from unknown or unverified sources.

Any edible labeled with a measure of weight and then "Psilocybin" next to it, such as "3.5g Psilocybin," is wrong, because this is actually how growers notate the weight of the fruiting body itself, rather than the psilocybin it contains. Pure Psilocybin is extremely cost-prohibitive to produce, and total psilocybin can vary widely from one batch to another. It's unlikely that you will see an accurate amount of psilocybin advertised.

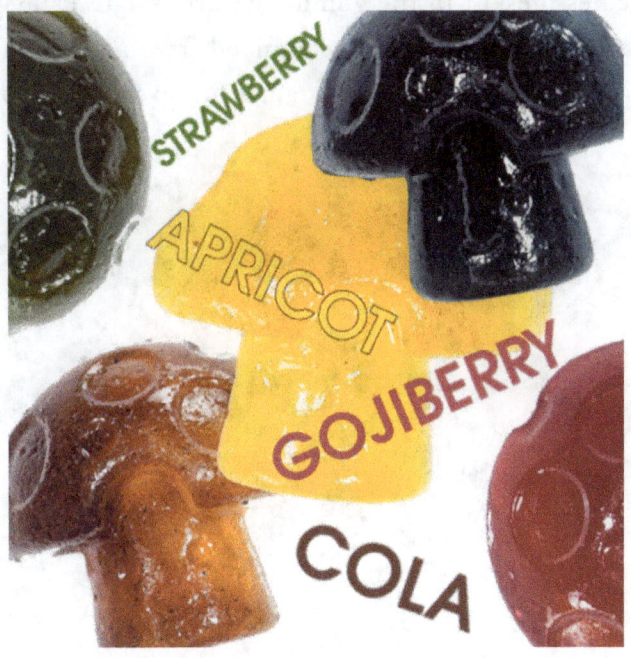

Magic Gummies: Mushroom powder or extracts are combined with a gelatin or pectin base, sweeteners, and flavorings to create gummies that are easy to consume and offer dose consistency. Gummies become the second most popular category of psychedelic edibles once extraction methods became popular. Each piece can be accurately dosed down to 500µg, and they taste just like the real thing, so please keep out of the reach of children.

The drawback to gummies is that the water that helps create the gelatin matrix promotes enzymatic activity. Oxygen molecules present in the gummy decarboxylate Psilocybin, causing it to degrade. We recommend freezing gummies in an airtight and light-proof container for up to three months.

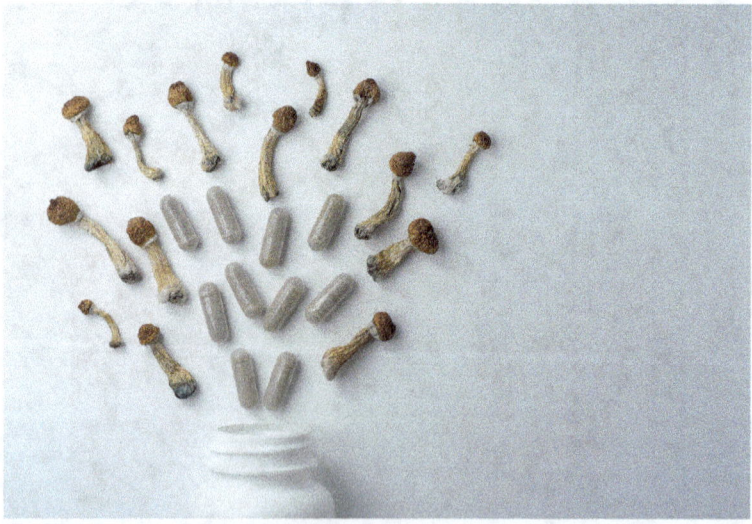

Capsules: Mushroom capsules offer a measured dosing option but can also pose similar risks as edibles. Verify the source and ensure the capsules contain pure, high-quality mushrooms.

Capsule sizes range from 000 (the largest) to 5 (the smallest), with some additional variations available. Here is a list of common capsule sizes:

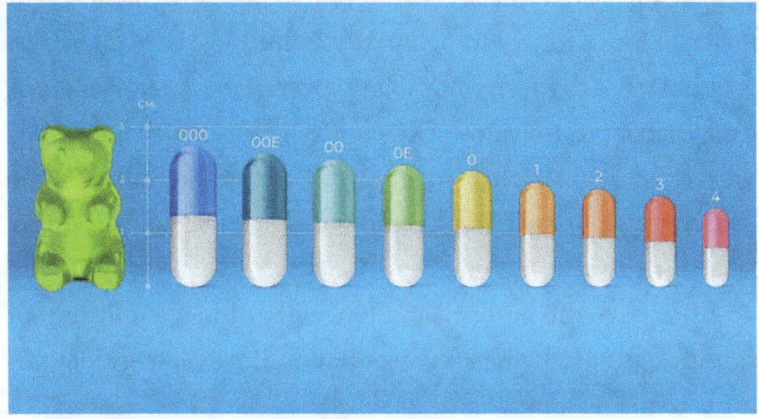

- 000—The largest standard size can hold about 800-1600 mg of powder.
- 00—A slightly smaller size, it can hold around 600-1100 mg of powder.
- 0—This size can hold approximately 400-800 mg of powder.
- 1—A smaller capsule with a capacity of around 300-600 mg of powder.
- 2—This size can hold approximately 200-400 mg of powder.
- 3—Even smaller, with a capacity of around 150-300 mg of powder.
- 4—A small capsule size, capable of holding around 120-240 mg of powder.

- 5—The smallest, with a capacity of approximately 60-130 mg of dry mushroom powder.

Capsules are typically made from gelatin or a plant-based material like hydroxypropyl methylcellulose (HPMC), which is important for those who follow vegetarian or vegan diets or have dietary restrictions. The choice of capsule size depends on factors such as the dosage of the active ingredients, the density of the powder or granules, and the Seeker's comfort level with swallowing medication.

To ensure the potency and longevity of magic mushroom capsules, proper storage is essential. Follow these guidelines to store magic mushroom capsules:

1. Keep them in an airtight container: Exposure to oxygen can cause the psilocybin to degrade over time. Using an airtight container, such as a glass jar with a tight-fitting lid or a vacuum-sealed bag, will help minimize oxygen exposure.
2. Store in a cool, dark place: Psilocybin is sensitive to heat and light, which can also cause it to break down. Storing the capsules in a cool, dark place, such as a cupboard or closet, will help maintain their potency.
3. Maintain a consistent temperature: Fluctuations in temperature can affect the quality of the capsules. Store them in an area with a stable temperature, away from heat sources, like radiators or direct sunlight.

4. Keep away from moisture: Moisture can cause the capsules to degrade and potentially develop mold. Ensure that the storage area is dry and consider using a desiccant packet (silica gel) in the container to absorb any excess moisture.

5. Avoid exposure to strong odors: Mushroom capsules can absorb odors from their surroundings, so store them away from sources of strong smells, such as spices or fragrant foods.

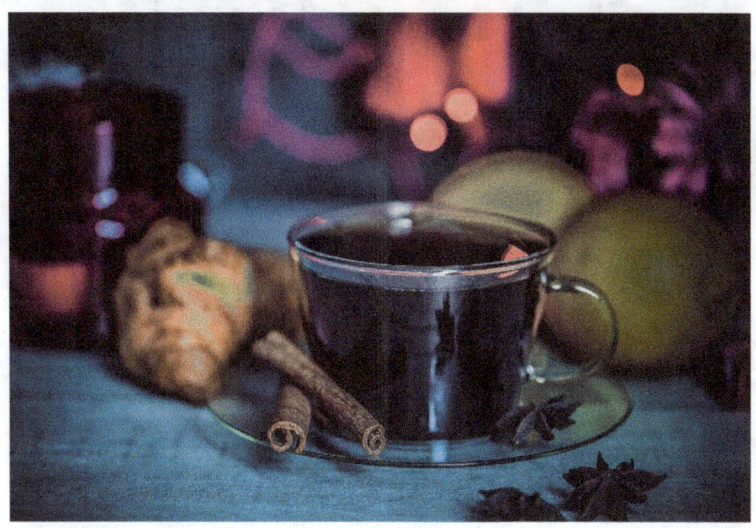

Magic Tea: Psilocybin mushrooms can be ground with a coffee grinder and steeped in hot water to create a tea, which is then strained and consumed. This method can help to mask the taste of the mushrooms and may lead to a quicker onset of the experience as the active compounds are more quickly absorbed by the body. The popular LemonTek involves steeping the juice of one lemon with ground mushrooms for thirty minutes to dephosphorylate the Psilocybin into Psilocin, which is the compound that crosses the blood/brain barrier. This technique does the work that your liver would if you consumed the active ingredients in a different way. The tea must be consumed within minutes before it degrades.

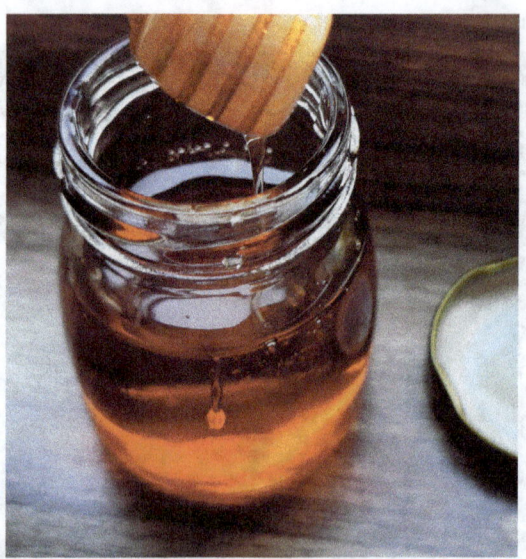

Magic honey: Psilocybin-infused honey is another edible option, and it is created by mixing coarsely ground mushrooms or Psilocybin extracts into honey. This mixture can be consumed on its own, added to tea or other beverages, or used as a sweetener in recipes.

CHAPTER 5

Sourcing Magic Mushrooms

Here, we delve into the multifaceted process of sourcing magic mushrooms, providing you with the essential knowledge to make informed decisions about obtaining these powerful fungi. We will discuss critical questions to ask your source, examine the role of religious organizations and psychedelic societies in connecting Seekers to magic mushrooms, explore the growing trend of mushroom retreats, and consider the option of cultivating your own psilocybin mushrooms.

By understanding these various avenues, you will be better equipped to embark on your journey of self-discovery and personal growth, confidently and responsibly.

5.1 Religious Organizations

Numerous religious organizations around the world integrate the use of psychedelic substances, including psilocybin mushrooms, into their spiritual practices. Participating in ceremonies or events hosted by these organizations can offer Seekers a safer and structured environment for exploring the effects of psilocybin. Some of these religious groups include:

- *Native American Church*: This organization primarily uses peyote, a cactus containing the psychedelic compound mescaline, as a sacrament in their ceremonies. However, some branches of the Native American Church have also been known to incorporate the use of psilocybin mushrooms, especially in regions where peyote is less accessible or abundant.
- *Neo-Shamanism*: Neo-shamanism is a contemporary spiritual movement that draws inspiration from the traditional practices of indigenous cultures worldwide. Some branches of neo-shamanism utilize plant-based entheogens, including psilocybin mushrooms, in their rituals and ceremonies. These gatherings are often led by experienced practitioners who guide participants through the psychedelic experience, fostering self-exploration and spiritual growth.
- *Psychedelic churches*: A growing number of modern churches and spiritual organizations have formed around the use of psychedelic substances as sacraments. These groups often emphasize the importance of intention, set and setting, and responsible use in their practices, and may include the use of psilocybin mushrooms in their ceremonies.

5.2 Psychedelic Societies

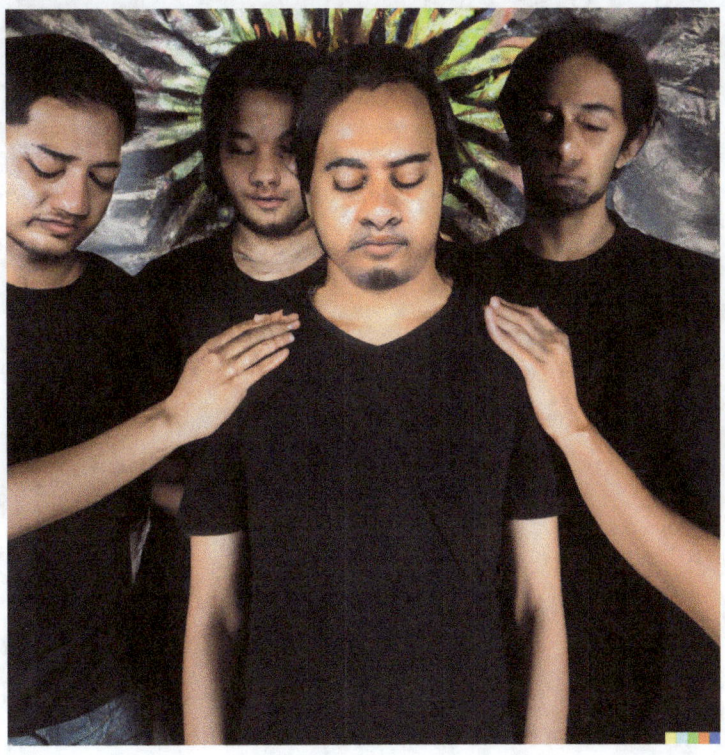

Psychedelic organizations or societies are dedicated to fostering understanding, responsible use, and appreciation for psychedelic substances such as psilocybin mushrooms. These groups can be valuable resources for those interested in learning more about sourcing and using psilocybin mushrooms safely, as they often provide the following opportunities and services:

- *Educational events*: Psychedelic societies frequently host lectures, panel discussions, and seminars that feature experts in the fields of psychedelic research, therapy, and policy. These events provide a wealth of information on various aspects of psilocybin use, including sourcing, safety precautions, and the latest scientific findings.
- *Workshops*: In addition to educational events, some societies offer workshops that focus on specific skills related to psychedelic use. These may include sessions on mushroom identification, cultivation, or harm reduction strategies.
- *Networking opportunities*: Attending events and gatherings organized by psychedelic societies can help you connect with experienced members and other like-minded individuals. These connections can be invaluable for obtaining reliable information, advice, and support on your psychedelic journey.
- *Online resources*: Many psychedelic societies maintain websites, blogs, or social media accounts that provide informative articles, research updates, and links to other resources related to psilocybin mushrooms and psychedelic use in general.
- *Support groups*: Some psychedelic societies host support groups or integration circles for individuals who have had challenging experiences or who are seeking guidance on incorporating insights from their psychedelic journeys into their daily lives.

To find a psychedelic association in your area, start by conducting an online search or reaching out to local organizations focused on mental health, spirituality, or alternative medicine. You can also explore national or international organizations, such as the Multidisciplinary Association for Psychedelic Studies (MAPS) or the The Entheology Project, which may have local chapters or affiliated groups in your region.

5.3 Mushroom Retreats

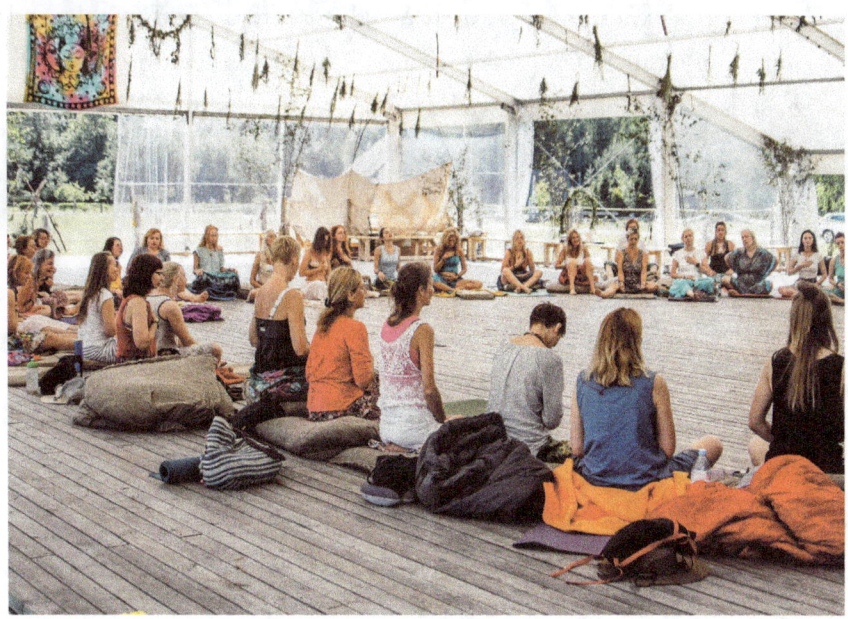

Psilocybin mushroom retreats provide a unique opportunity for individuals seeking a secure, guided, and therapeutic environment for their psychedelic journey. These retreats are typically held in countries where psilocybin mushrooms are legal or decriminalized, and are facilitated by trained professionals who prioritize safety and responsible use.

Some key features and benefits of attending a psilocybin mushroom retreat include:

1. *Professional facilitation*: Psilocybin retreats are led by experienced guides or therapists who can offer support and guidance throughout a Seeker's experience. They can help create a comfortable and nurturing atmosphere, assist with navigating challenging emotions or sensations, and ensure well-being during the retreat.

2. *Safe and legal environment*: By choosing a retreat in a country where psilocybin mushrooms are legal or decriminalized, you can minimize the risks associated with obtaining and using these substances. Additionally, retreat facilitators typically source their mushrooms from reliable suppliers, meaning that the materials consumed are safe and trustworthy.

3. Structured experience: Psilocybin retreats often include a carefully curated program of activities designed to enhance your experience and facilitate personal growth. These may involve preparatory workshops, guided meditations, breathwork sessions, or group sharing circles.

4. *Integration support*: A crucial aspect of the psychedelic journey is integrating the insights and emotions encountered during the experience. Psilocybin retreats often provide post-session support

through group discussions, one-on-one counseling, or follow-up resources to help you process and apply what you have learned.

5. *Community connection*: Attending a retreat allows you to connect with like-minded individuals who share your interest in personal growth and self-exploration. These connections can provide ongoing support and encouragement as you continue your journey.

By attending a professionally organized psilocybin mushroom retreat, you can embark on a transformative journey within a secure, guided, and therapeutic environment, maximizing the potential benefits and minimizing risks associated with psychedelic experiences.

5.4: Professional Facilitators

A facilitator or guide is a trained professional who can help you have a safe and positive experience with magic mushrooms. They can provide guidance and support during your journey, and help you to integrate your experiences into your everyday life. Engaging a facilitator can be especially beneficial for first-time Seekers or those seeking deeper self-exploration.

Reasons to consider using a facilitator for your magic mushroom experience include:

1. *Preparation and education*: Facilitators can help you prepare for your experience by providing information about magic mushrooms,

dosage, and potential effects. They can also educate you about best practices for ensuring a safe and positive experience.

2. *Creating a safe environment*: A facilitator will work to create a supportive atmosphere that promotes relaxation and introspection. This may involve setting up a comfortable space, curating calming music or visuals, and using techniques such as guided meditation or breathwork.

3. *Guidance through challenging experiences*: If you encounter difficult emotions or sensations during your journey, a facilitator can provide reassurance, grounding techniques, or simply a comforting presence to help you navigate the experience with greater ease.

4. *Integration support*: After your experience, a facilitator can assist you in processing and integrating the insights and emotions you've encountered. This may involve discussing your journey, offering suggestions for further self-reflection, or providing resources for ongoing personal growth.

If you are interested in finding a qualified facilitator, consider the following steps:

- *Research*: Look for facilitators with experience and training in psychedelic therapy or guidance. This may involve searching online, attending workshops, or joining psychedelic community forums.
- *Credentials and testimonials*: Seek out facilitators with verified credentials and positive testimonials from previous clients. This can provide reassurance that they are skilled and trustworthy.
- *Personal connection*: Schedule a consultation or interview with potential facilitators to discuss your goals, expectations, and

any concerns you may have. This will allow you to gauge whether you feel comfortable and supported by the individual.

- By taking the time to find a skilled and compassionate facilitator, you can enhance the safety, depth, and overall quality of your magic mushroom experience.

5.5 Growing Mushrooms

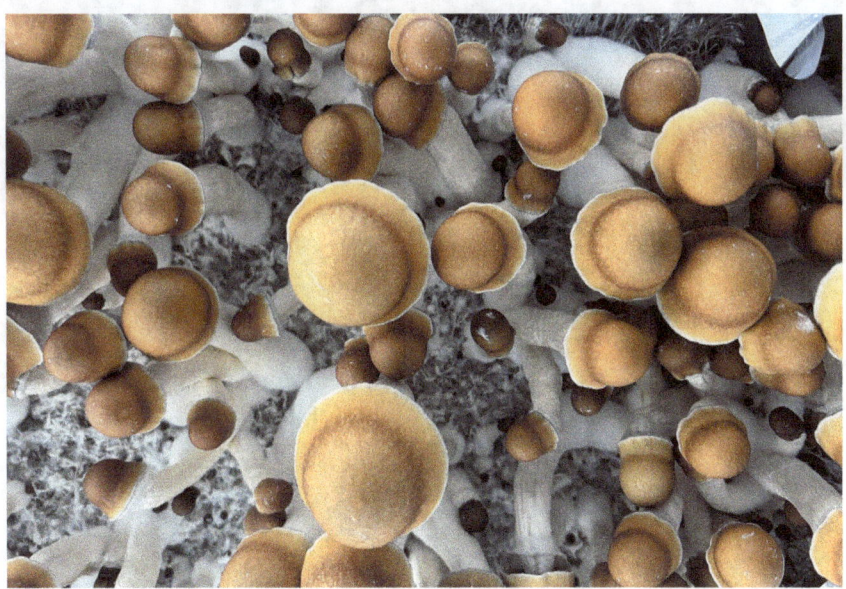

This is a monotub of Ol' Dirty Penis Envy (ODPE), ready for harvest.

Growing your own magic mushrooms can be a rewarding and cost-effective way to obtain them for personal use. However, it is important to note that the cultivation of Psilocybin-containing mushrooms is illegal in many parts of the world. It is essential to research the laws in your area before attempting to grow your own.

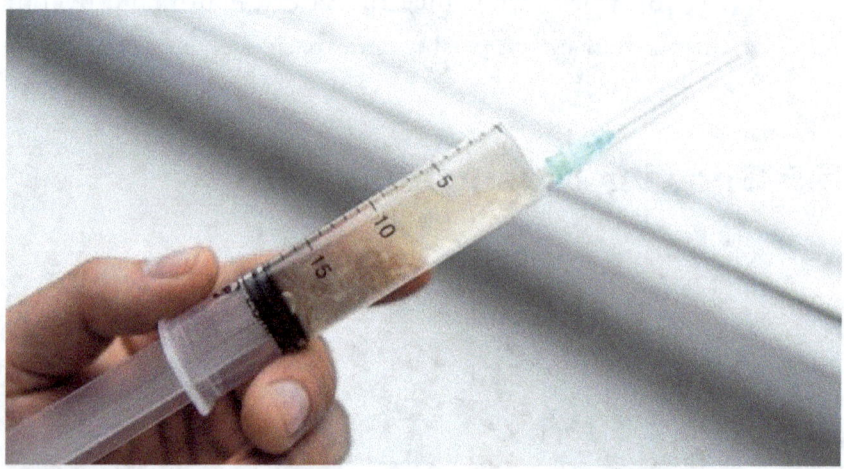

The most popular and easiest way to grow your own magic mushrooms at home involves the use of grow kits and spore syringes. These kits usually contain all the materials you need to grow mushrooms, including the spores or mycelium, substrate, a tub, and instructions for use.

Assuming that growing your own magic mushrooms is legal where you live, the process involves several steps:

1. *Obtaining spores*: Spores are the microscopic reproductive cells of mushrooms. You can purchase spores online from a reputable vendor.
2. *Creating a growing environment*: Magic mushrooms can be grown in a variety of environments, but the most common method

involves introducing the spores into a sterilized substrate, such as a mixture of vermiculite and brown rice flour, in a container like a jar or a plastic bag.

3. *Inoculating the substrate*: Once the substrate is prepared, the spores are injected into the jar or bag using a sterile syringe.

4. *Incubation*: The inoculated substrate is then kept in a warm, dark place for a period of several weeks to allow the mycelium—the vegetative part of the fungus—to colonize the substrate.

5. *Fruiting*: After the mycelium has colonized the substrate, the fruiting process begins. Home growers must expose the substrate to light and humidity to stimulate the growth of mushrooms.

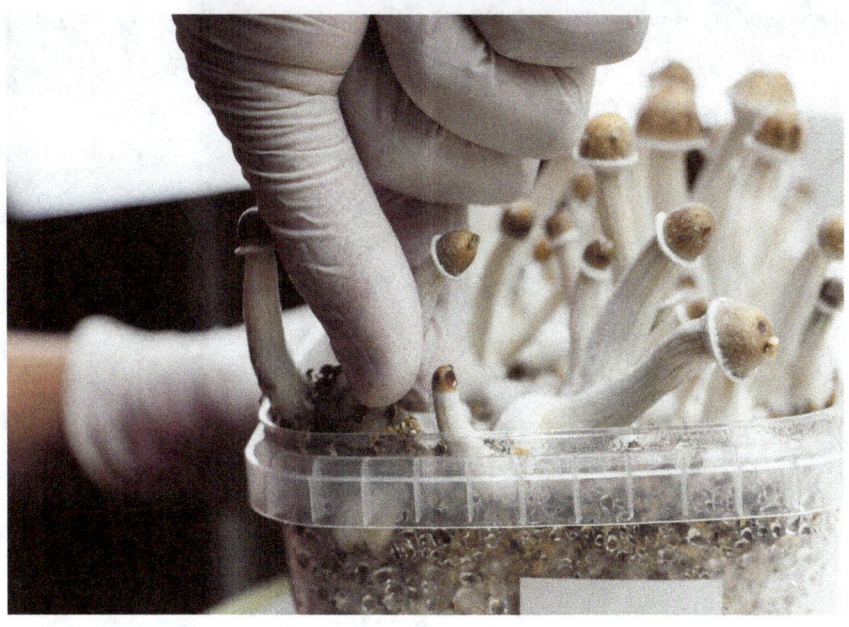

It is important to follow proper hygiene and sterilization protocols throughout the process to avoid contamination and ensure safe and healthy mushroom growth. Mold and contamination are major issues that can render an otherwise healthy tub unusable.

Even if you feel confident about your supplies and process, it is crucial to use caution and responsibility when consuming any Psilocybin-containing mushrooms, regardless of whether they were purchased or grown at home.

When sourcing Psilocybin mushrooms, it's essential to prioritize safety and reliability. By thoroughly researching your options, verifying the quality and legality of the mushrooms, and considering more structured sources like religious organizations, psychedelic societies, or mushroom retreats, you can minimize risks and maximize the potential for a positive, transformative experience.

Always exercise caution, and remember that your safety and well-being are of the utmost importance on your journey with Psilocybin mushrooms.

5.6 Questions to Ask Your Source

When engaging with an mushroom cultivator or processor, ask the right questions to ensure product safety, quality, and transparency. Here are some questions you may want to consider asking:

1. What strains of mushrooms do you cultivate or process? Most mushrooms are the psilocybe cubensis variety.

2. What growing techniques do you use? Ensure that the mushrooms are grown in a sanitary environment and that the proper growing conditions for the species are met.

3. Are your mushrooms organic? Organically grown mushrooms are less likely to be contaminated with pesticides or other chemicals.

4. How are the mushrooms processed? Ensure that the mushrooms are processed and handled in a sanitary manner and that the processing facility follows proper food safety protocols

5. Can you provide lab testing results for your mushrooms? Look for mushrooms that have been tested for contaminants, such as heavy metals or bacteria.

6. What is the expiration date of the product? Look for fresh mushrooms that have a reasonable shelf life.

7. How to they store their mushrooms? Mushrooms are extremely water loving and degrade rapidly in the presence of moisture. They should be vacuum sealed with a desiccant pack and kept frozen to preserve the psilocybin.

8. How do you ensure consistent potency and dosage in your products? Consistent dosing is crucial for a safe and enjoyable experience. Ask the manufacturer about their quality control measures and testing protocols to ensure uniformity across their products.

9. What extraction method do you use for the psychoactive compounds? Different extraction methods can impact the purity and potency of the final product. Knowing a supplier's extraction process can give you insights into the quality of the edibles they produce.

10. Do you try to follow Good Manufacturing Practices (GMP)? GMP compliance means that a manufacturer has agreed to adhere to strict guidelines that ensure the quality, safety, and consistency of their products. There is no official Psychedelic GMP standard as of now, but any supplier should always strive for the highest standards.

11. How do you handle product recalls or customer complaints? Do you provide support by email, SMS, or phone? Understanding the manufacturer's approach to customer questions and concerns can give you insights into their commitment to customer satisfaction and product safety.

12. How do you ensure the freshness of your products? How do you determine shelf life? Ask about the manufacturer's packaging, storage, and shipping methods. All of these factors play a role in the edibles remaining fresh, stable, and potent.

CHAPTER 6

Set, Setting and Intention

Set, setting, and intention are some of the key concepts that are important to consider when using psilocybin or other psychedelics. The more mushrooms you consume, the more important the set, setting and intention become. They are the internal and external factors that influence a "trip." Set refers to the mental and emotional state of the person taking the substance. It includes factors such as their expectations, past experiences, and mental health.

A positive set can contribute to a more beneficial experience

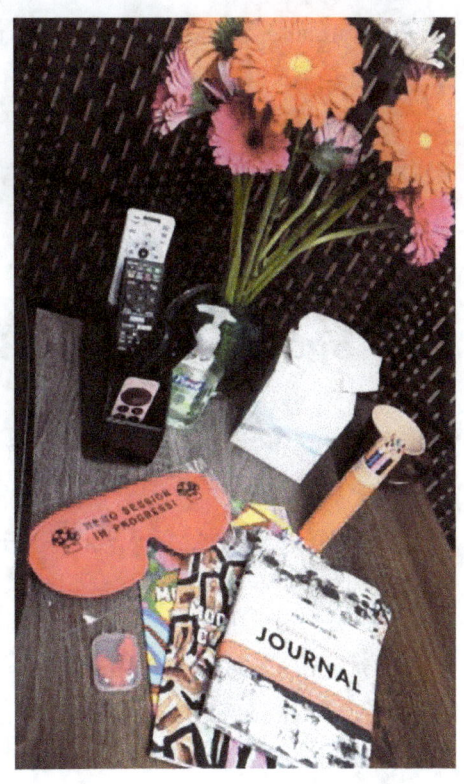

and outcome while a negative set can hinder it. Setting refers to the physical and social environment in which the experience takes place. It requires a safe, comfortable, and supportive environment that can facilitate the experience in a positive direction.

The setting can include factors such as lighting, sound, and people involved. Intention refers to the purpose or goal of the experience. It helps the person taking the substance to set their intentions, expectations, and desired outcomes of the experience.

Having a clear intention can promote a positive set and provide a sense of guidance and direction during the experience. All three concepts (set, setting, and intention) are crucial to consider when engaging in a psilocybin or other psychedelic experience. Proper preparation, including setting a positive intention and creating a supportive and safe setting, can improve the likelihood of a positive experience and long-term benefits.

6.1 Negative Set and Setting

While some individuals may choose to use psychedelics in social settings like clubs, parties, or concerts, these environments can present potential risks and challenges. Inappropriate settings may:

1. Be overstimulating, with loud music, bright lights, and large crowds, all of which could potentially cause anxiety or sensory overload.
2. Lack privacy or personal space, making it difficult to process emotions or thoughts during the experience.

3. Offer limited access to a quiet, safe space to retreat to if the experience becomes overwhelming or uncomfortable.
4. Be filled with unfamiliar people or distractions that could negatively influence your mindset and experience.

6.2 Positive Set and Setting

When using psychedelic substances in the 2g-5g range, certain minor factors can have a significant impact on your overall experience. By choosing a familiar and comfortable environment, such as your home or a close friend's place, you can help create a calm and relaxing atmosphere that is conducive to a positive experience. It's also important to minimize distractions and set aside ample time for the experience and recovery. You can prepare the space with comfortable seating, soft lighting, and calming decorations like artwork or plants, as well as curate a playlist of calming, inspiring, or meaningful music to help set a relaxing and positive tone. Pleasant scents such as essential oils or incense can also help create a calming ambiance. Engaging in meditation or mindfulness exercises before the journey can help you cultivate a calm and focused mindset, which can be helpful during the experience. By taking these steps to create a supportive set and setting, you can help ensure a safe, positive, and transformative experience with psychedelic substances.

Nature can be an ideal setting for a hero's journey (a term that refers to a high-dose psychedelic experience that can be challenging but transformative). Being surrounded by trees, mountains, rivers, and animals can inspire a deep connection with the natural world and provide a sense of awe and wonder that can be very helpful during a high-dose psilocybin experience. However, it's important to choose a safe and comfortable location in nature and be prepared for any weather conditions or unexpected events that may arise. It's also recommended to have an experienced guide or facilitator to help navigate the experience. Remember that set and setting are crucial factors, and what is best for one person may not work for another.

Meditation or mindfulness exercises can be helpful in cultivating a calm and focused mindset before a mushroom journey. These practices can help you reduce anxiety and anxious thoughts, increase self-awareness, and promote a feeling of calm and relaxation. Here are some tips that may help: 1. Find a quiet and comfortable place where you can sit without interruption for a period of time. 2. Set a timer for five to ten minutes. Start with a short duration and gradually increase over time. 3. Sit comfortably but upright. You can sit on a cushion or a chair. Allow your body to relax, but try to maintain an alert and upright posture. 4. Focus your attention on your breath. Notice the sensations of your breath, such as the rise and fall of your chest or the sensation of air moving in and out of your nostrils. 5. As you focus on your breath, you may notice that thoughts come up. This is normal and expected. When thoughts come up, acknowledge them and gently bring your attention back to your breath. 6. As you practice this exercise regularly, you may find that you become more aware of your thoughts and emotions throughout the day and that you can more easily direct your attention where you choose. With regular practice, meditation or mindfulness exercises can be helpful in creating a calm and focused mindset that can support a positive experience during a mushroom journey. It's important to note that the practice of meditation or mindfulness may not completely eliminate all anxious or challenging thoughts and emotions, but it can help you create a more grounded and centered mindset that can support you in navigating the experience.

- Choose a familiar, comfortable, and calming environment, such as your home or a close friend's place.
- Minimize distractions by turning off electronic devices, informing those around you of your plans, and setting aside ample time for the experience and recovery.
- Prepare the space with comfortable seating, soft lighting, and calming decorations like artwork or plants.
- Curate a playlist of calming, inspiring, or meaningful music, and have pleasant scents available, such as essential oils or incense.

6.2.1 A Comfortable and Calming Space

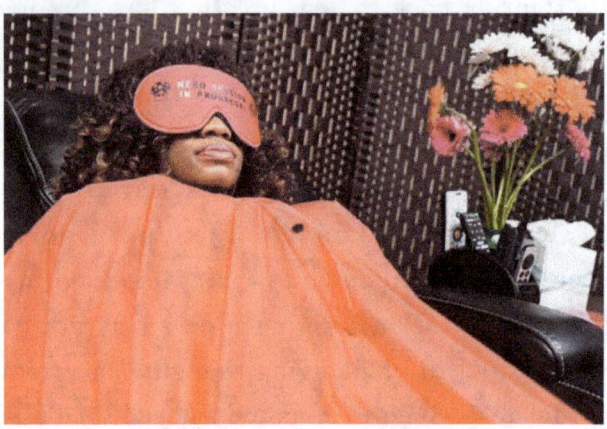

Ensure your surroundings are clean, clutter-free, and arranged in a way that makes you feel at ease. Consider using sensory management products like a body sock for added comfort and security. Surround yourself with soft blankets, cushions, and objects that evoke positive feelings.

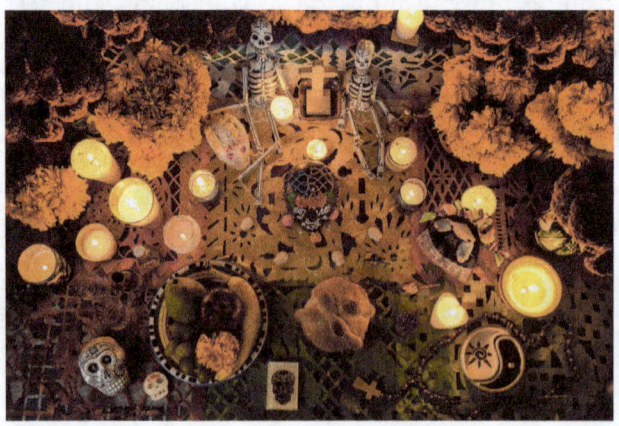

Choose music that is calming or inspiring, depending on your preferences. For those who like silence, use ear-plugs to block out any unwanted noises. Set the lighting to a level that feels soothing; you might want to use dimmed lights or candles to create a warm ambiance. Introduce pleasant scents using essential oils or incense that help you relax and enhance your experience.

Moreover, without proper preparation, set, and setting, people who consume magic mushrooms without intention or a sense of responsibility can find themselves overwhelmed by the intensity of the experience. They may be unable to process the insights and emotions that arise, leading to distress or confusion. This can lead to negative outcomes such as anxiety, panic attacks, and even the emergence of mental illness or psychotic episodes, in rare cases.

6.2.2 Mindfulness Exercises

6.2.2.1 Body Scan

This exercise involves lying down or sitting comfortably and focusing on each part of your body, starting from your toes and moving intentionally and slowly all the way to the top of your head. As you focus on each part, notice any sensations, thoughts, or emotions that come up without judgment or analysis.

6.2.2.2 Breath Awareness

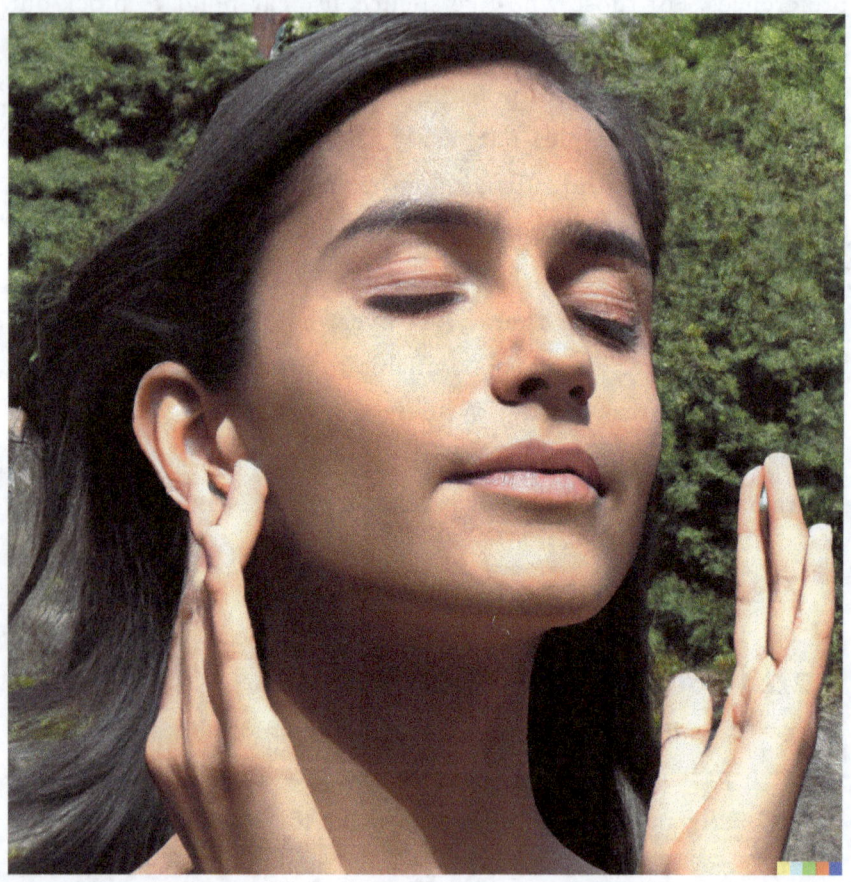

Sit comfortably with your eyes closed and focus on your breath. Notice the sensation of the breath as it enters and exits your nostrils or mouth and of your body breathing. If your mind wanders, gently bring it back to the breath.

6.2.2.3 Loving-Kindness Meditation

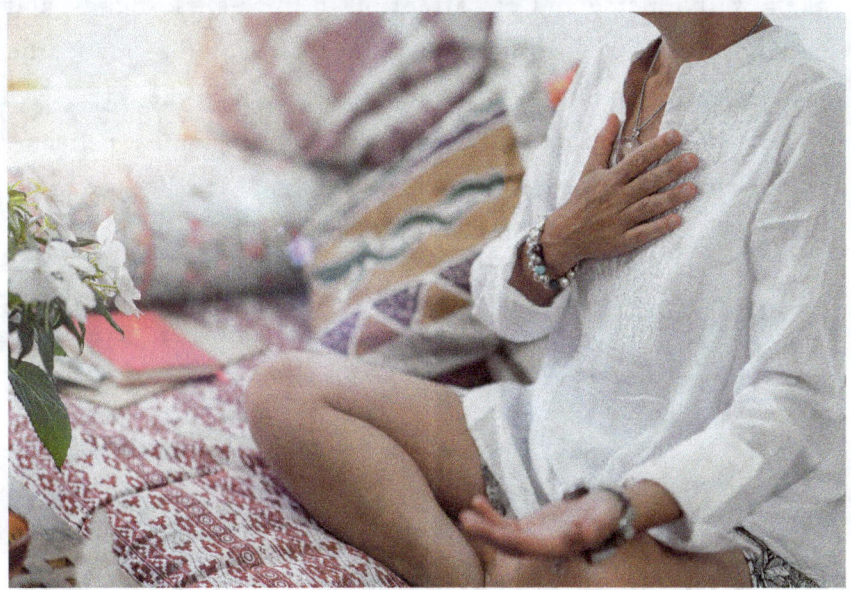

This practice involves directing love and kindness towards yourself and others. Start by sitting comfortably and focusing on your breath. Then repeat mantras such as "May I be happy," "May I be healthy," "May I be safe," and so on.

6.2.2.4 Gratitude Practice

Take a few minutes each day to reflect on the things you're grateful for. It could be something as simple as the warmth of the sun or the sound of birds chirping. Focus on the feeling of gratitude in your body.

6.2.2.5 Mindful Walking

Take a walk outside and pay attention to the sights, sounds, and sensations around you. Notice how your feet feel on the ground, the sound of leaves rustling in the wind, or the colors of the sky.

Remember, mindfulness is a skill that requires practice, patience, and persistence. The more you do it, the easier it will become to achieve a deeper presence in your everyday life.

6.3: Intention

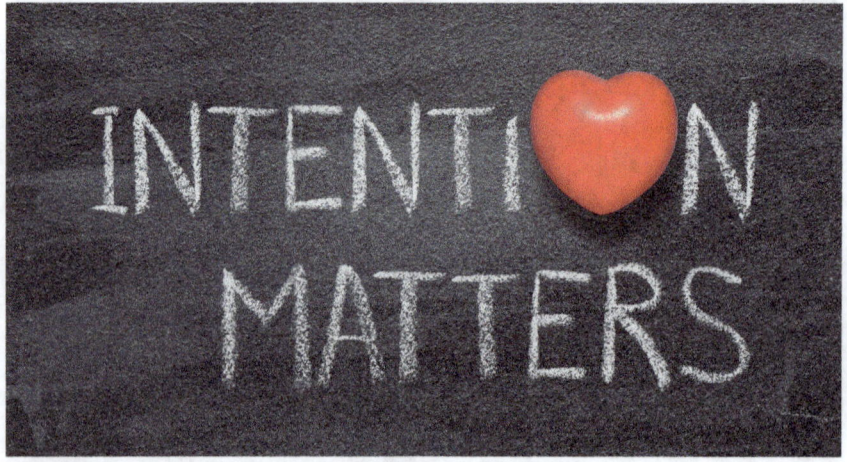

When it comes to an experience with psilocybin mushrooms, setting a clear intention prior to starting the journey can have a profound impact on the experience. Setting the intention is essentially defining and verbalizing what you are hoping to gain or discover from the experience. This could be anything from a deeper understanding of yourself or the world around you to an intention to overcome a specific fear or challenge. The act of setting a clear intention can give purpose to your experience and help you feel more in control of it. It can also guide the trajectory of the experience and serve as a roadmap as you navigate through it. By having a clear intention in mind, you may find that you have a greater sense of clarity and focus during the experience, which can help you extract more meaning and insight from it. Intention setting can also serve as a grounding tool during moments of confusion or fear. It can help bring you back to a sense of purpose and provide perspective and a sense of direction when the experience feels overwhelming or chaotic. In addition to setting the intention, it can also be helpful to hold it close throughout the experience, reminding yourself of it regularly and using it as a tool for reflection and guidance. Overall, setting a clear intention before the journey can make a significant impact on the experience, giving it purpose and direction and helping you extract greater meaning and insights. By taking the time to define your intentions, you can set the stage for a transformative and meaningful journey.

Please approach the use of magic mushrooms with respect, intention, and caution. When used appropriately and with the proper guidance, Psilocybin mushrooms can be a powerful tool for personal growth and healing.

When people consume magic mushrooms primarily for a recreational or perceptual experience, they risk missing out on the transformative potential of these substances. The mind-altering effects of Psilocybin mushrooms can be powerful, and, if these active compounds are taken improperly or without intention, their use lead to negative consequences. Some people may become fixated on the perceptual aspects of the experience and seek out higher and higher doses. To do so could miss some important points along the way.

6.3.1 Types of Intentions

The setting of intentions before a psilocybin journey can take many forms, depending on what the individual hopes to achieve or experience. Different types of intentions are available for setting and there is no one right way of doing it.

Different types of intentions can be used to set the tone for a psilocybin journey that reflects the individual's objectives, motivations, and questions. While setting intentions is beneficial, individuals must also keep an open mind and hold the right attitude to ensure they get the most of their experience.

The following are common types of intentions that individuals can use:

1. *Personal growth*: This type of intention is characterized by seeking self-improvement or developing specific skills. These could be related to personal development goals such as learning a new skill or achieving a particular goal in an area of one's life.
2. *Emotional healing*: This type of intention focuses on addressing unresolved emotions or past traumas. The intention can be set to confront guilt, shame, fear, anger, anxiety, or depression that is causing emotional and mental distress.

3. *Spiritual exploration*: This type of intention is designed to connect with a higher power or explore one's spirituality. The intention can be to gain greater clarity and insight into one's spirituality or to find meaning and purpose in one's life.

4. *Creativity enhancement*: This type of intention is focused on unlocking creative potential or overcoming creative blocks. When creativity blocks exist, the intention may be set to to find inspirations or to remove fear and self-doubt that may deter creativity.

5. *Relationship improvement*: This type of intention focuses on fostering deeper connections with others or improving communication skills. The intention can be to improve one's connections with family, friends, and coworkers or to address and resolve relationship difficulties.

6.3.2 Formulating Your Intention

Formulating your intention is an essential component of preparing for a psychedelic journey. By creating a clear and meaningful intention, you are putting yourself in the best possible position to make the most out of the experience, gain valuable insights, and achieve the growth or change you seek. Here are some steps to help you create a meaningful intention:

1. *Reflect on your current life situation*: Before you begin, take some time to reflect on your current life situation. What areas of your

life do you feel need growth or change? Are there any unresolved issues, worries, or negative patterns that you want to address? Reflecting on these questions can help you clarify your intentions and what you hope to get out of the experience.

2. *Be specific*: Once you have identified areas of growth and change, it's essential to be specific about what you hope to achieve or learn from the experience. For example, if you're struggling with anxiety, you may want to set the intention to explore the root causes of your anxiety and find ways to manage it more effectively. Alternatively, if you're looking to gain insight into your relationships, you may set the intention to look inward and reflect on where you may be contributing to any problems in those relationships.

3. *Write down your intention*: Writing down your intention can help solidify it in your mind. By putting it in writing, you are making a commitment to yourself and setting a clear goal for the journey.

4. *Share your intention with a trusted friend*: Sharing your intention with a trusted friend or trip-sitter can be helpful for added accountability. When you articulate your intention to someone else, you are making a public declaration of your goals, which can help motivate and inspire you to stay on track. Remember, the intention you set is crucial and should be tailored to your specific needs and goals.

Take time to reflect and articulate your goals, then commit to them fully. With a clear and meaningful intention in place, you will be better equipped to navigate the experience, gain valuable insights, and achieve the growth or change you seek.

6.3.3 Set an Intention!

Here are a few examples of setting productive intentions prior to a psychedelic hero journey:

1. *Letting go of negative emotions*: Before embarking on the journey, set the intention to release any negative emotions or feelings that have been weighing you down. By letting go of these emotions, you can free up mental space to explore new perspectives and insights.
2. *Overcoming anxiety*: If anxiety is a persistent problem for you, set the intention to address it during your journey. Focus on accepting your feelings and gaining a more nuanced understanding of their root causes. This could lead to breakthroughs in managing anxiety in your daily life
3. *Seeking spiritual guidance*: Set the intention to explore your spiritual beliefs or gain guidance from higher powers during the journey. By adopting a mindset of openness, you may gain unique insights into your spirituality and unlock previously unknown aspects of your consciousness
4. *Healing from past traumas*: If you have experienced past traumas, set the intention to address them during your journey. Focus on accepting and healing from those traumas, using the experience to gain new perspectives and breaking free from their influence in your life.

5. *Enhancing creativity*: Set the intention to explore new artistic directions or embrace creativity in your life. By opening up to new perspectives and possibilities, you may be able to unlock a new level of creative potential that was previously hidden.

6.3.4 Keep Going!

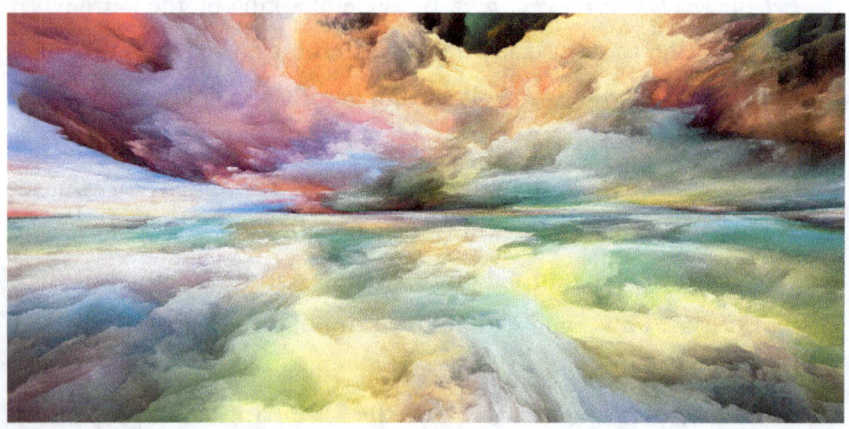

In the Hero's Journey, the main character encounters various challenges and obstacles that test their courage, strength, and wisdom. Similarly, during a psychedelic journey, the Seeker may encounter difficult or uncomfortable experiences that test their patience and ability to let go of expectations. After setting an intention for the journey, it's important to remain patient and open-minded to allow the next phases of the journey to continue. The journey may have uncomfortable moments, such as confronting past traumas or difficult emotions, and it's important to be patient and allow these experiences to unfold without resistance.

Patience is also necessary because the insights and growth gained from a psychedelic journey may not come immediately. It may take some time to process and integrate the insights gained during the journey into everyday life. Like the next phases of the Hero's Journey, the next phases of a psychedelic journey require patience and perseverance to face new challenges and continue the process of growth and transformation.

It's important to remain patient and open-minded to allow the next phases of the journey to unfold, even if they may be difficult or uncomfortable. The insights gained from the journey may require further patience and perseverance to fully integrate into everyday life and continue the process of growth and transformation.

CHAPTER 7

The Experience

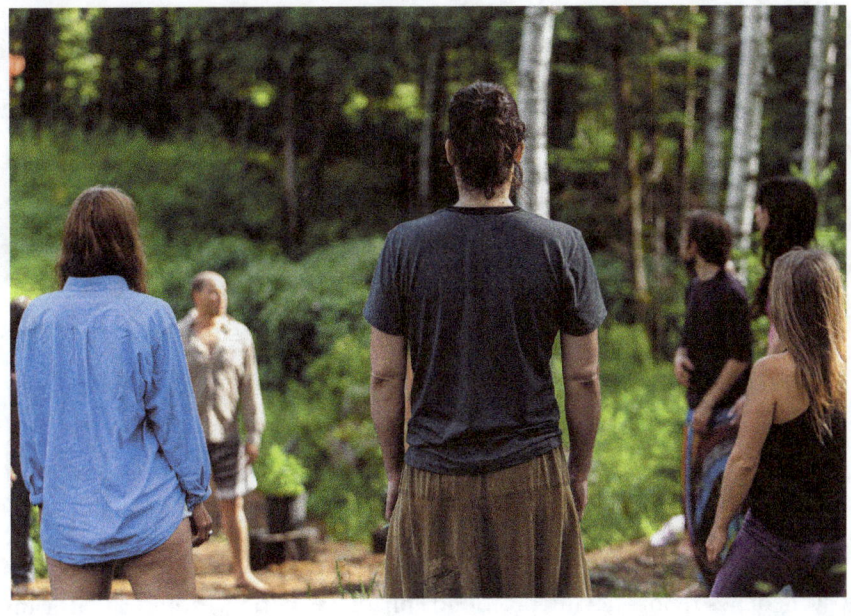

Psychedelic "trips" can be profound, transformative, and deeply meaningful. However, they can also be challenging and potentially risky if not approached with proper preparation, intention, and guidance. If you are planning to consume magic mushrooms, it's important to take certain precautions and set yourself up for a safe and positive experience. In this section, we will provide some recommendations to help you prepare for your journey and make the most out of your experience with Psilocybin mushrooms.

7.1 The Significance of Rituals

Rituals play a significant role in psychedelic settings. The traditional use of psychedelic plants almost always involves ritual. Ritual is the stylized expression of belief. It provides a "sacred" space within which the Mystery can manifest, a template for its expression in terms understandable to humans. It therefore doesn't matter what the ritual is, as long as what emerges from it is comprehensible to you. Rituals can help to create a safe and supportive environment for the psychedelic experience. They can provide a sense of structure and predictability, which can be comforting for individuals who may feel anxious or uncertain about the experience. Rituals can also help to set intentions and create a sense of purpose for the psychedelic journey. In addition, rituals can help to facilitate a connection with the divine or spiritual realm. Many individuals who use psychedelics report having profound spiritual experiences, and rituals can help to create a container for these experiences to occur. Overall, rituals can be a powerful tool for individuals who are using psychedelics for spiritual or therapeutic purposes. They can help to create a supportive and meaningful environment for the experience, and can facilitate a deeper connection with the self, others, and the divine.

Traditional contexts: Indigenous cultures have used psychedelics for centuries in the context of religious and spiritual practices and have developed extensive rituals around their use. For example, in the Mazatec culture of Oaxaca, Mexico, indigenous people have been using mushrooms in religious ceremonies for generations. Maria Sabina, a Mazatec healer, became well-known for her use of mushrooms in her healing ceremonies, which involved a specific ritual with the sacred mushroom. The ceremony usually takes place at night, with a fire lit in the center of a circular hut. Participants sit around the fire, forming a circle, and Sabina or another leader begins by invoking the spirits and asking for guidance and healing. Once the spirits are invoked, Sabina would administer the mushrooms to the participants. During the experience, participants are encouraged to close their eyes and listen to the music, which is an essential component of the ceremony. Some participants will chant or sing, and others may remain silent. As the psychoactive effects of the mushrooms begin, the participants often report a sense of awe, connectedness to nature and the spirit realm, and often report receiving messages from spirits or ancestors. Following the ceremony, participants may share their experiences with the group, and Sabina or another leader will interpret their experiences and offer guidance. The Mazatec ceremony is just one example of the importance of ritual in psychedelic use among Indigenous cultures. These rituals are carefully crafted around the specific needs and goals of the community, emphasizing the importance of connection to nature, spirits, and ancestors. They foster a sense of safety and intentionality in the psychedelic experience and provide a sacred space for the exploration of the self and the universe. Indigenous cultures have recognized the importance of ritual in psychedelic use for centuries, and with the growing interest in psychedelic therapy and open use among other groups, it is essential that these traditions and practices be acknowledged, respected, and preserved.

Modern contexts: While psychedelic use has been part of human culture for centuries, contemporary psychedelic Seekers have adapted and developed their own ways of using these substances to maximize their therapeutic benefits. One significant way they have done this is through the development of rituals. Rituals can provide structure and a sense of intentionality, which can be beneficial for enhancing the psychedelic experience and providing a safe container for healing. This is especially crucial in the context of psychedelic therapy where a skilled practitioner will help guide patients through a structured session that includes an intentional setting, music, eye shades, and even massage or other forms of touch. For many contemporary Seekers, the ritual begins before the psychedelic experience itself. They may fast, meditate or engage in other activities for several days prior to their "trip", to help cleanse and prepare their mind and body. The use of intention setting and affirmations are also common, where the Seeker takes time to set clear goals for their experience and focus on the desired outcomes. During the experience, the ritual may include the use of sacred objects, such as crystals or feathers, playing particular music or choosing a particular art to guide their experience, or engaging with nature. Attention to their immediate environment, such as dimming lights, lighting candles, or burning sage to cleanse the space, further enhances the sense of intention and focus.

After the experience, ritual can help Seekers integrate their insights and revelations from the "trip" through journaling, meditation, or sharing their experience with others. This can further embed the lessons learned during the experience, allowing them to make lasting changes and personal growth. By developing their own rituals, contemporary Seekers are able to foster a sense of safety and intentionality in their psychedelic experiences, emphasizing their potential for healing and growth. By creating a structured approach, they are able to better navigate the often-challenging and disorienting nature of psychedelic journeys.

7.2 Designing Your Ceremony

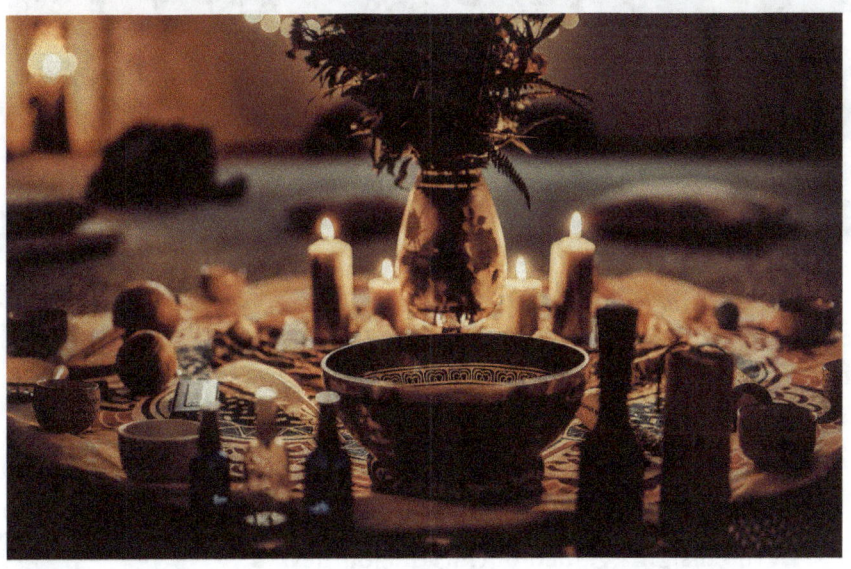

- *The Psilocybin Tea/Chocolate Ceremony*: Involves the mindful preparation and consumption of Psilocybin-infused tea or unfermented cacao, accompanied by meditation, chanting, or prayer.

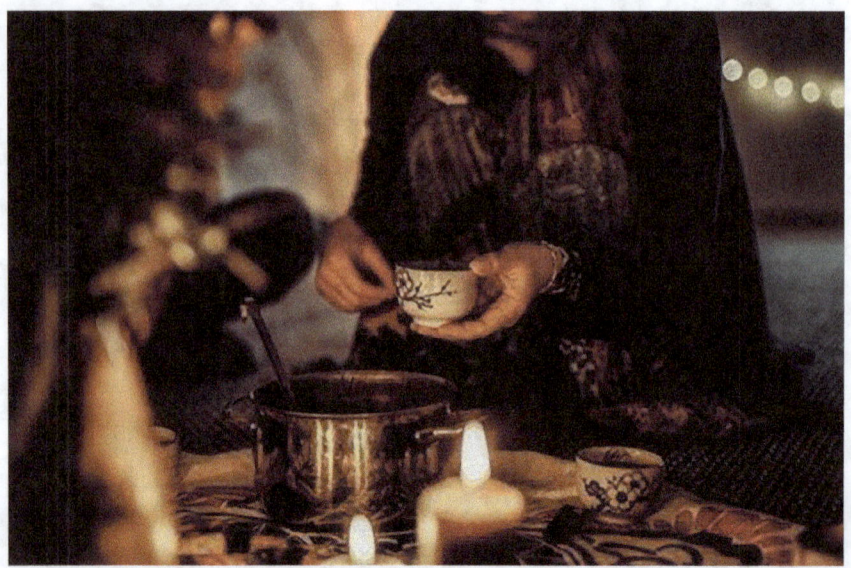

Developing a ritual can deepen your psychedelic experience and create a sense of sacredness.

- *Shamanic Drumming Journey*: Incorporates rhythmic drumming or rattling to induce a trance-like state, allowing for deep introspection and exploration.
- *Mandala Creation*: Engages in the artistic process of creating a mandala, a symbolic representation of the universe, to express the insights gained during the journey.

By participating in a unique ceremony that aligns with your intentions and resonates with your beliefs, you can establish a deeper connection to your inner self and enhance the overall impact of your journey.

Remember to remain open and flexible, as the experience may reveal new insights or directions that can further inform and enrich your ritual practice.

7.3 Beginning the Experience

When planning to take a dose of Psilocybin, there are several factors to consider for a positive and beneficial experience. In this section, we will discuss the best practices for consuming Psilocybin, including whether or not to eat beforehand, staying hydrated, avoiding competing substances, and understanding the duration of effects of their potential "trip."

7.3.1 Empty Stomach or No?

It's generally recommended to consume Psilocybin mushrooms on an empty stomach, as this can help to reduce the likelihood of nausea and enhance absorption of the active compounds. However, eating a light meal a few hours before ingestion may help to provide a base for the stomach and prevent feelings of lightheadedness or weakness. Avoid heavy or greasy foods, as they can slow down the absorption of Psilocybin and may contribute to feelings of discomfort.

Taking something acidic with magic mushrooms is thought to help enhance the effects of psilocybin by converting it to its more active form, psilocin. Psilocin is a relatively unstable molecule that breaks down quickly in alkaline conditions, so consuming something acidic can help stabilize it and increase its bioavailability. This is why some people recommend taking magic mushrooms with lemon juice, vinegar, or other acidic foods or drinks. Some examples of acidic foods or drinks that can be consumed with magic mushrooms include citrus fruits, cranberry juice, and apple cider vinegar. It is important to note that while taking your dose with an acidic food or liquid can enhance the effects of the mushrooms, it can also increase the intensity of the experience, so Seekers should exercise caution when determining dosage.

7.3.2 Hydration

Avoid drinking too much water when taking active mushrooms as the oxygen molecule will oxidize the alkaloids more quickly. Staying well-hydrated before and after taking your dose is important, as water helps to support bodily functions and maintain a sense of well-being. Make sure to drink water throughout the experience to prevent dehydration, which can exacerbate feelings of discomfort or disorientation.

7.3.3 Timing and Duration of Effects

It typically takes between thirty minutes to one hour for the effects to become noticeable after consuming Psilocybin. The peak of the experience usually occurs around two to four hours after ingestion, and the overall effects can last between four to eight hours, depending on factors such as the dose, individual sensitivity, and the form in which Psilocybin was consumed.

It is crucial to set aside ample time for the "trip," including time for the come-up, peak, and comedown phases, as well as additional time afterward to rest and reflect on what happened during the journey. Avoid scheduling any important or potentially stressful activities on the day of your Psilocybin session to ensure a comfortable and relaxed mindset. You might want to also earmark the day after, as there can be lingering effects.

By following these guidelines, you can prepare for a Psilocybin experience that is safe, comfortable, and conducive to personal growth or healing. Remember that individual experiences will vary, and it's essential to listen to your body and adjust your approach as needed.

CHAPTER 8

The Importance of Integration

Properly integrating your psychedelic experience is vital for translating the insights gained on the journey into lasting life changes. The efficacy of integration comes down to personal courage and readiness. You have to be willing to do the work because, after all, this is therapy! The mind is the critical limiting factor.

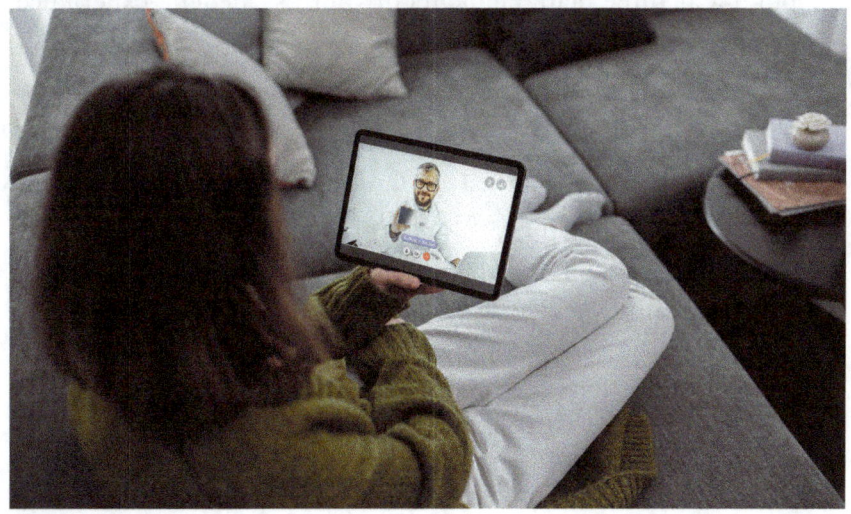

8.1 Reflection and Self-assessment

Reflection and self-assessment are crucial elements of psychedelic integration as they provide an opportunity to process and make meaning of the experience. Here are some methods you can use to reflect on your experience:

1. Guided meditation: Guided meditations are designed to help you focus your awareness and to cultivate a meditative state. A guided meditation designed for integration after a psychedelic experience can be a powerful tool for processing your insights and emotions. It can help you access a deeper level of reflection, and provide an opportunity to connect with your inner wisdom.

2. Three-Pillar Reflection: This method of reflection involves looking at three main elements of your psychedelic experience. The first pillar is the insights that you gained during your journey. This could be philosophical realizations, a new perspective on an old issue, or spiritual revelations. The second pillar is the emotions that you experienced during your journey. This could include intense feelings of love, joy, fear, sadness, or confusion. Finally, the third pillar is the actions that you can take in response to the insights and emotions you experienced. This may involve changes in behavior, re-prioritizing aspects of your life, or simply living with greater awareness.

3. Journaling: Writing can be a powerful way to reflect on your experience, as it allows you to put your thoughts and feelings

down on paper. You can write about the insights and emotions that arose during your journey, what you learned, any challenges you faced, and the actions you plan to take in response.

Talking with a therapist or integration coach: Working with a licensed therapist or integration coach can be a beneficial option for processing a psychedelic experience. They can help you understand and work through any difficult emotions or insights that arose during the journey and can provide guidance as you integrate the experience into your life. Overall, reflection and self-assessment are essential for successful psychedelic integration. These practices can help you make sense of your experience, deepen your understanding, and offer opportunities for growth and transformation.

8.2 Process Your Experience

Processing your psychedelic experience is a critical part of integration, as it helps you make sense of the often-profound insights and emotions that may arise during your journey. Here are some questions to help guide your reflection and processing:

- What were the most significant insights or realizations you had during your journey? Psychedelic experiences are often accompanied by profound insights and realizations that might change your worldview. Take time to reflect on the insights or realizations that resonated with you the most during your journey. Write them down and spend time reflecting on how they could affect your life.

- How did your emotions change throughout the experience, and what did you learn about yourself through these emotions? Psychedelics often bring up intense emotions. Reflect on what emotions you experienced during the journey, and how they changed throughout. Take note of the emotions that were difficult to navigate and those that felt positive and useful. Reflect on how these emotions are attached to particular processes within yourself.

- What aspects of your life might benefit from the application of these insights? After reflecting on your insights and emotions, think about how they can be translated into usable steps in your everyday life. Ask yourself what aspects of your life you can apply these insights and emotions to, such as your relationships, career, or wellbeing. Consider what changes you might need to make in your life in order to honor these insights.

Taking the time to process your experience is an essential part of integration as it helps you to maximize the benefits of the journey and incorporate its lessons into your daily life. Combine the above-mentioned questions with other reflection techniques like journaling, talking with trusted friends or professionals, and creative expression. By sitting with your experience and allowing yourself time to reflect and integrate, you can find meaning, purpose, and growth.

8.3 Incorporating Lessons Into Daily Life

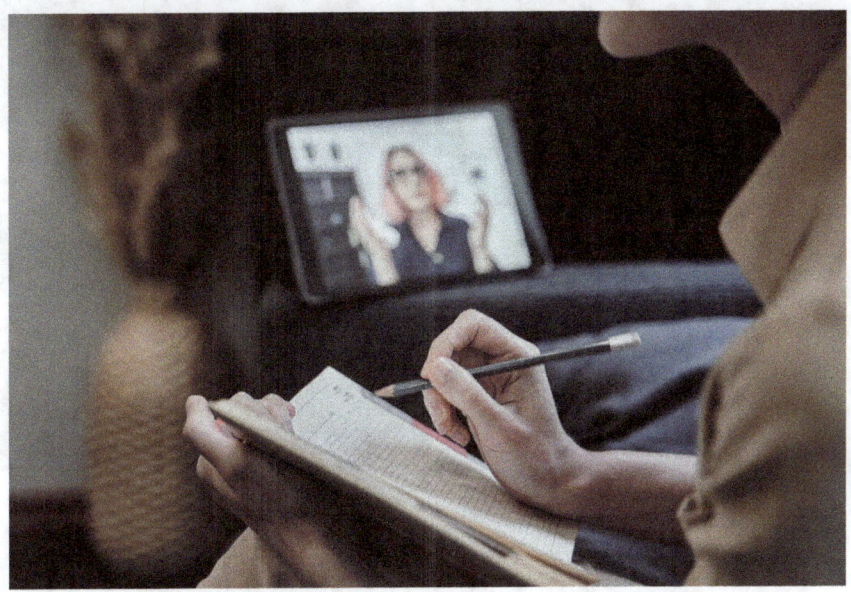

Once you have started to process the insights you've gained post-trip, take the time to develop a personal action plan that outlines specific steps you can take to apply these insights into your life in practical terms. This could include changes to habits, relationships, a situation that has been bothering you, or refinements made to short- or long-term personal goals.

1. Create a daily or weekly reminder to revisit your insights and check in on your progress, ensuring that you maintain focus on your personal growth.

2. Incorporate breathwork techniques into your integration process. Breathwork can help calm the mind and release any residual tension or emotions from your journey.
3. Share your experience with trusted friends or family members who can provide understanding, encouragement, and accountability.
4. Join a psychedelic integration support group, either in-person or online, to connect with others who have had similar experiences and can offer guidance and camaraderie.
5. Consider working with a professional facilitator who can help guide you through the integration process and provide additional resources and support.

Remember, integration is a process that takes time and effort. It's important to be patient with yourself and celebrate your progress as it comes, without forcing it. By actively working to integrate your experience, you can make meaningful changes in your life and continue on your journey of self-discovery.

When you take a psychedelic journey, it offers a unique opportunity for transformation and personal growth. However, the transformation and personal growth are only possible when you commit yourself to integration and learning from your experience. By committing yourself to the integration process after the psychedelic experience, you can understand the insights and messages it brought to you. You can also adopt new perspectives and uncover specific things you need to work on to improve your life quality. Through the integration process, you can make sense of your insights, visions, or messages. You can also identify ways to apply the lessons you've learned to your daily life. This way, your psychedelic experience can become an integral part of your personal growth that helps you move towards positive change in your life. It is essential to commit to the integration process and work on the insights brought by the experience to derive the maximum possible benefits from it.

CHAPTER 9

Be the Hero!

9.1 Summing Up Your Experience

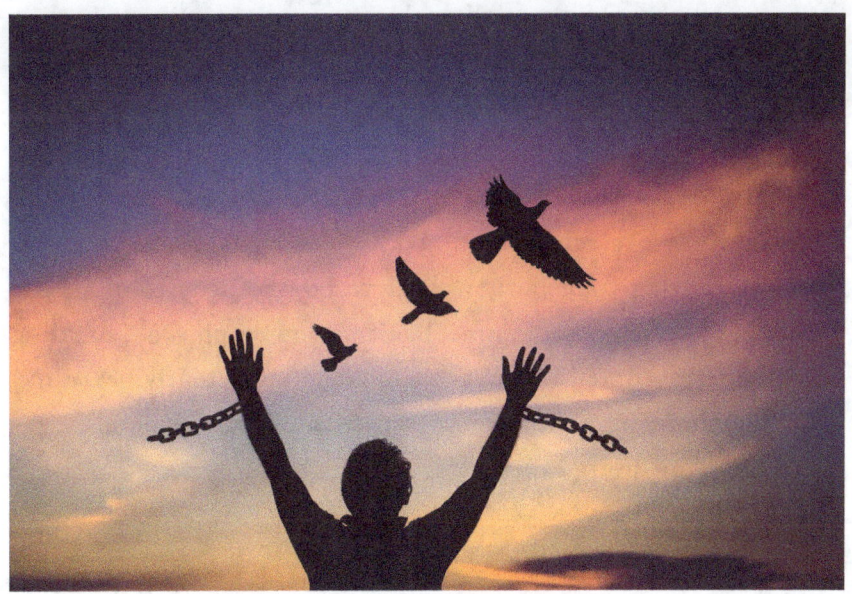

Reflecting on the experience as a whole and acknowledging the progress you've made is essential to well-being!

9.1.1 How Well Were Your Intentions Met?

Take time to revisit the goals and intentions you set before embarking on your Psilocybin journey. Assess whether these intentions were fulfilled, or if certain areas may require further exploration. Consider how your experience aligned with your expectations and what aspects of your journey were particularly meaningful.

9.1.2 What Were the Highlights?

Reflect on any profound insights, emotional breakthroughs, or transformative moments that you experienced during your journey. Contemplate how these revelations can be integrated into your daily life and what changes you might make as a result. Identifying specific actions or practices to implement these insights can help promote lasting personal growth.

9.1.3 How Did You Overcome Challenges?

Recognize any obstacles, emotional hurdles, or trying experiences that arose during your journey. Analyze how you confronted these challenges and what coping mechanisms you employed, including how well they worked or what you might do differently next time. Learning from these moments can cultivate resilience and better prepare you for future experiences.

9.2 Experience Self-discovery and Growth Daily

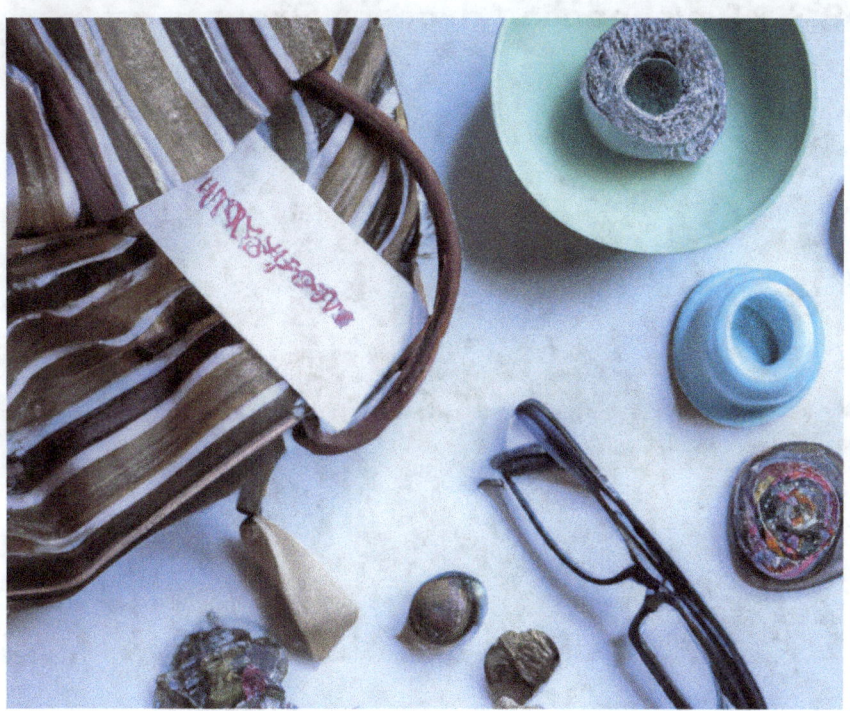

9.3 Get Involved!

9.3.1 Psychedelic Conferences or Events

Stay connected with the broader psychedelic community by participating in conferences, workshops, or online forums. These gatherings and groups can offer valuable insights, foster connections with like-minded individuals, and provide opportunities for continued learning.

9.3.2 Psychedelic Advocacy Groups

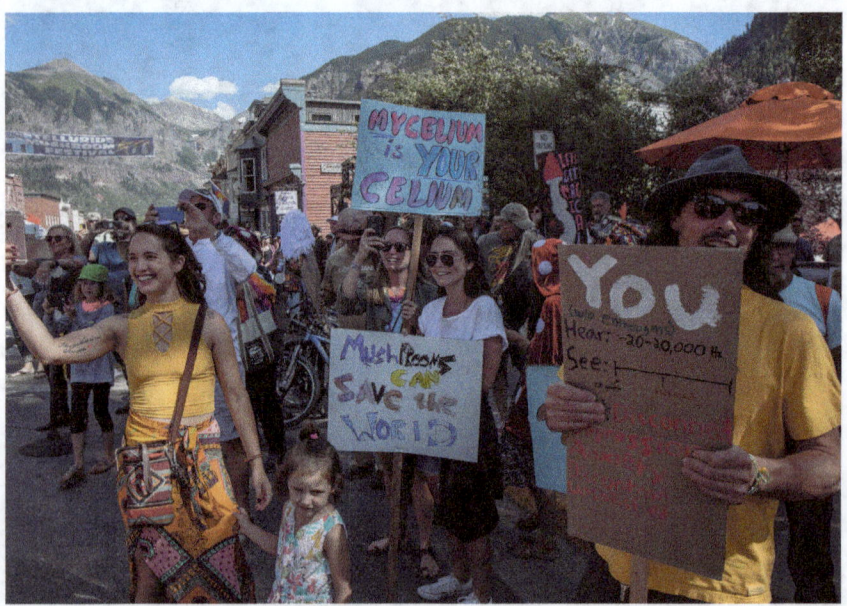

There are several psychedelic advocacy groups out there, and getting involved with them can be an excellent way to stay informed about the latest developments in the field. These organizations dedicate their efforts to advocating for psychedelic research, policy reform, and education. By participating in these groups, you will learn from like-minded individuals who are passionate about entheogens. You will also gain access to valuable resources, including scientific studies, literature, and discussions on psychedelic use. With this knowledge, you will be better informed to participate in meaningful dialogue about the relative harms and merits of psychedelics. Some advocacy groups have local chapters that hold regular meetings and events, while others are online communities. A few examples of psychedelic advocacy groups include The Entheology Project, Multidisciplinary Association for Psychedelic Studies (MAPS), The Beckley Foundation, Students for Sensible Drug Policy (SSDP), and The Psychedelic Science Review. Participating in these groups can provide you with a supportive community that shares your interests, along with opportunities to make a positive impact in the entheogenic community.

9.3.3 Connect With Like-minded People

Connecting with like-minded people who share your interest in psychedelics can provide a supportive community that can be beneficial in your integration process. Engaging with people who have gone through similar experiences may allow you to discuss the insights you gained during your journey, which can help you gain better clarity and understanding of them. This can be especially useful when you are struggling to comprehend how the experience can help you in your personal growth. By sharing your experiences with similarly interested people, you can also gain different perspectives and learn ways to apply the lessons learned to your daily life. Additionally, meeting and building relationships with people who share your interests and values can be an enriching experience in itself, fostering a sense of community and belonging. There are different ways to connect with people who share your interest in psychedelics. For example, attending a local meetup or joining online communities such as Reddit and Facebook groups can provide you with an opportunity to interact and engage with a community of people. By actively participating in these groups, asking and answering questions, and sharing your experiences, you can build relationships with similar-minded people. Another way to meet like-minded people is by attending events such as conferences, concerts, or festivals that focus on psychedelic culture. These events can be a great way to mingle with people who share your interests and forge lasting relationships. Overall, connecting with like-minded people can be an essential part of the integration process, providing you with social support, new perspectives, and a sense of belonging to a broader community.

CHAPTER 10

Be Happy!

It's important to remember that Psilocybin is a powerful substance that should be treated with respect and caution. Please be conservative while experimenting with psychedelics and consult with a trained facilitator or integrator before dabbling or deepening your commitment to the journey.

Throughout this guide, we have explored the history, science, and potential therapeutic applications of Psilocybin, as well as the legal and social landscape surrounding its use. A growing body of research has catalogued the promising benefits of Psilocybin-assisted therapy for various mental health conditions, and these developments have sparked a renewed global interest in this naturally occurring compound.

Despite the inconsistency between Psilocybin's legal status and its emerging therapeutic potential, there is a growing movement advocating for policy reform, increased research, and public education. These efforts aim to address the stigma associated with Psilocybin and facilitate the integration of Psilocybin-assisted therapy into mainstream mental health care.

As we move forward, it is crucial to continue supporting rigorous research on Psilocybin's safety, efficacy, and potential applications, as well as fostering open dialogue and education about its therapeutic possibilities. By doing so, we can better understand the potential of Psilocybin to revolutionize mental health care and provide innovative and effective treatments for those in need.

It is essential to remember that, while Psilocybin may offer promising therapeutic benefits, it is still a powerful substance that should be used with caution and under the guidance of trained professionals. This guide is intended to provide information and insight but should not replace the advice of a qualified healthcare provider.

As we navigate the future of Psilocybin and mental health care, let us approach this topic with curiosity, compassion, and a commitment to expanding our understanding for the betterment of all those who may benefit from this remarkable compound.

BRAIN TEASERS & PUZZLES!

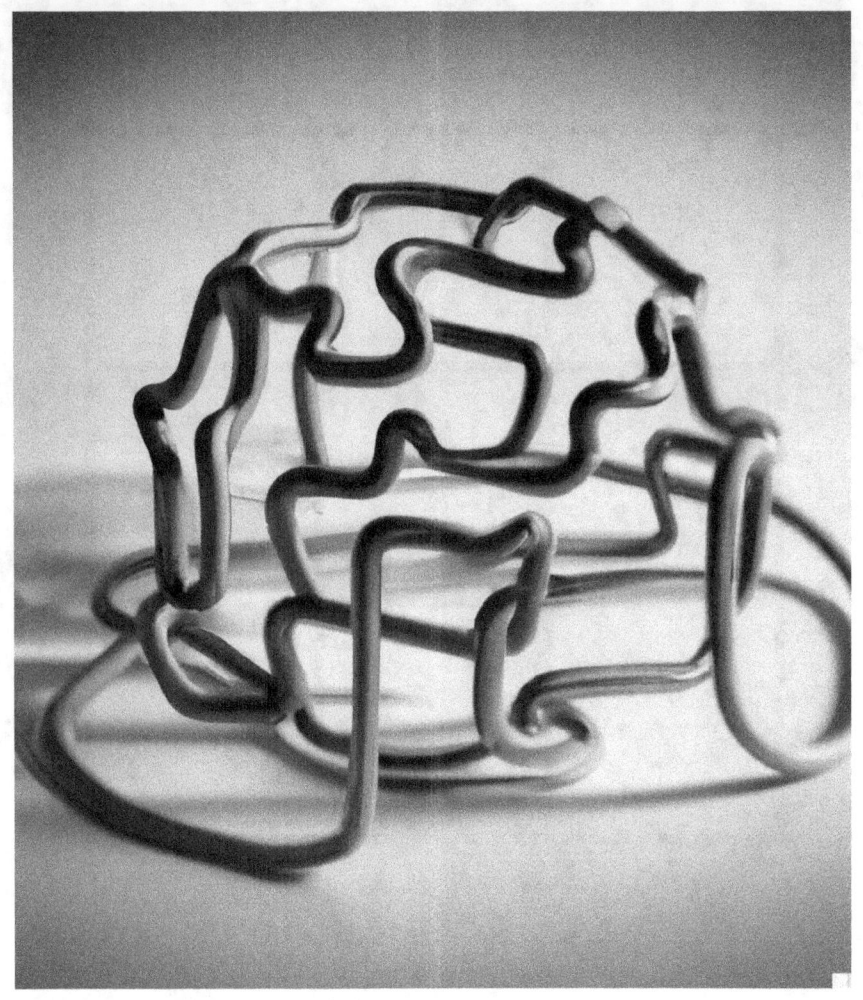

Here are some fun exercises to keep you safe and happy on the day of your "trip." Make sure your bags are packed with engaging activities designed to stimulate your mind and support your self-discovery journey!

Magic Square

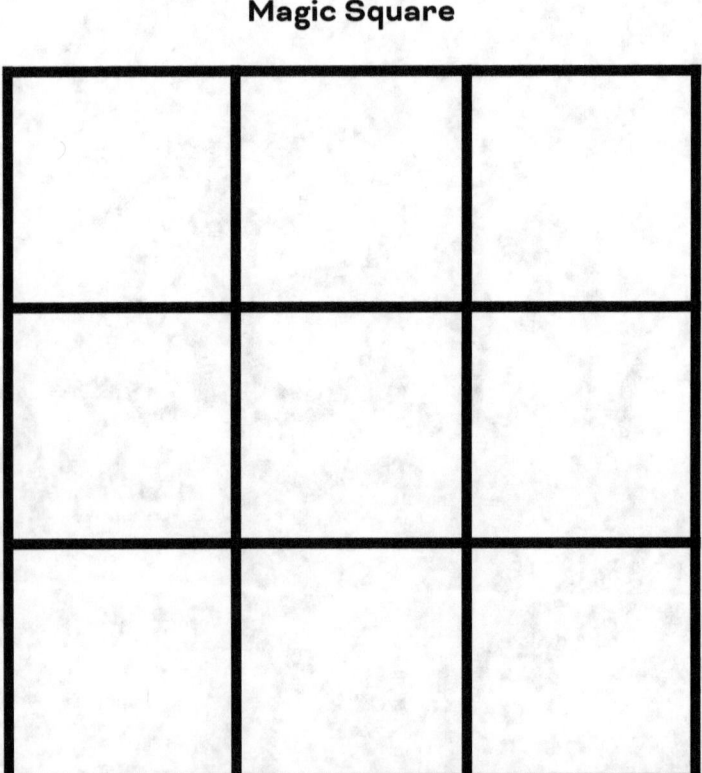

Fill in the empty cells with numbers 1 to 9 so that each row, column, and diagonal sums to the same number.

The Mushroom Conundrum

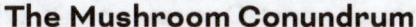

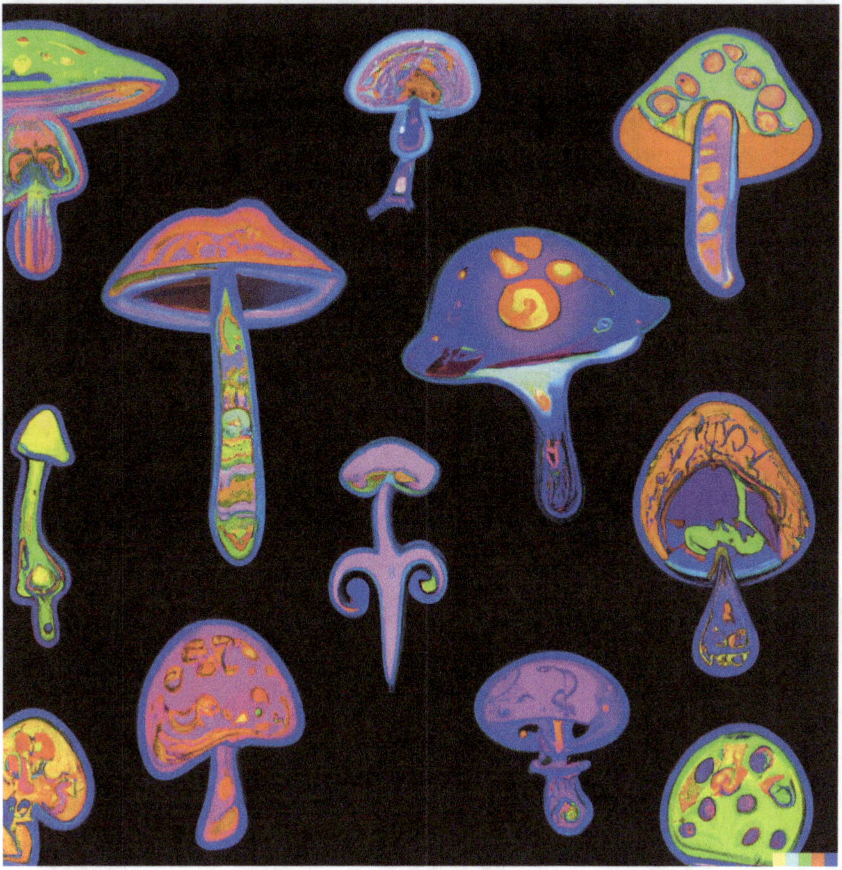

If you have eight mushrooms and you take away five, how many mushrooms do you have left? Now, imagine that each mushroom represents a different aspect of your life. What might these aspects be?

Entheogenic Crossword Puzzle

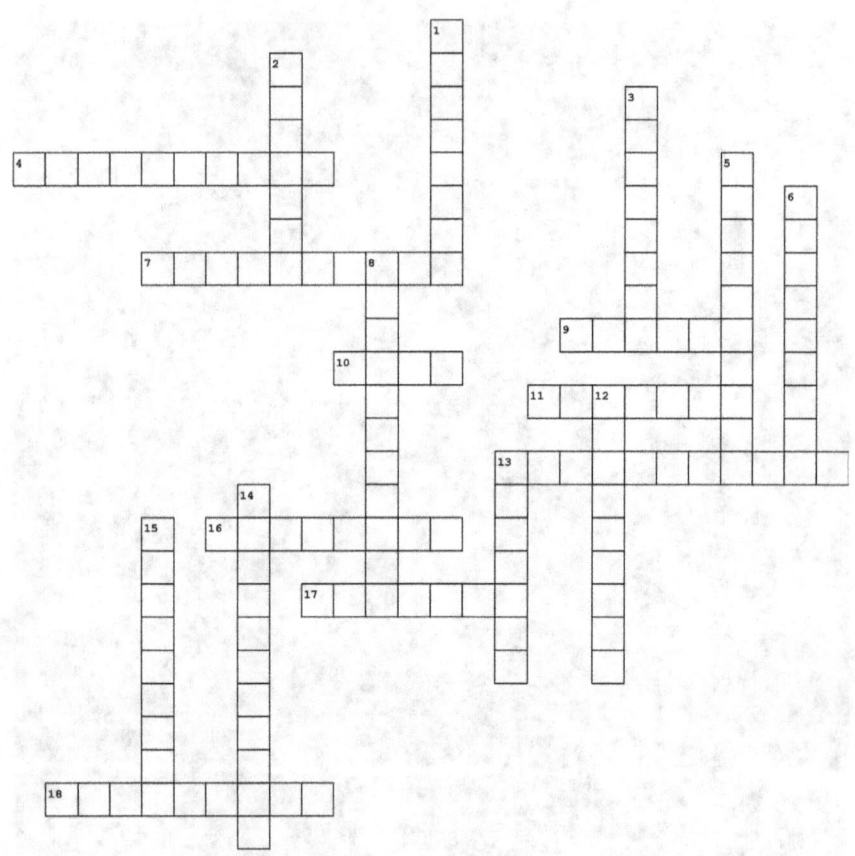

Across

4. The primary psychoactive compound found in magic mushrooms

7. A practice of focused concentration and relaxation used to cultivate mindfulness and self-awareness

9. The amount of Psilocybin consumed during a trip

10. Someone who has taken a large dose of magic mushrooms intended for intense, transformative experiences

11. Hallucinations experienced during a psychedelic trip

13. Taking a sub-threshold dose of a psychedelic for therapeutic or creative purposes

16. The vegetative part of the mushroom that grows underground

17. The mental state or attitude a person has before and during a psychedelic trip

18. A transformative experience characterized by a shift in consciousness and perspective

Down

1. The metabolite of Psilocybin responsible for its psychoactive effects

2. A profound realization or understanding gained during a psychedelic journey

3. Sclerotia that contain Psilocybin and are used as a substitute for magic mushrooms

5. One of the most common species of magic mushrooms found in the world

6. A substance used for spiritual or religious purposes

8. The process of incorporating insights from a psychedelic experience into daily life

12. The neurotransmitter that Psilocybin interacts with in the brain

13. Indigenous people of Mexico known for their traditional use of magic mushrooms during spiritual ceremonies

14. The experience of mixing sensory perceptions, such as hearing colors or seeing sounds

15. A reoccurrence of psychedelic effects after the initial trip has ended

Answer Bank

Awakening • Dosage • Entheogen • Flashback • Hero •
Insight • Integration • Mazatec • Meditation • Microdosing
• Mindset • Mycelium • P.Cubensis • Psilocin • Psilocybin •
Serotonin • Synesthesia • Truffles • Visuals

Magic Coloring

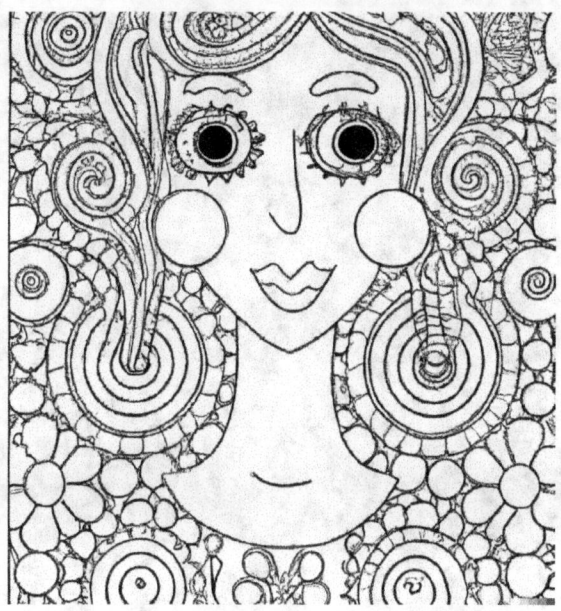

Gather your coloring supplies, such as colored pencils, markers, or crayons. Start by taking a few deep breaths and focusing on the present moment. Let go of any worries or distractions. Begin coloring this image, starting with a color that appeals to you. Focus on the sensation of the coloring instrument in your hand, and the movement of your hand across the page. Pay attention to the colors you choose and how they interact with each other. Take your time, and don't worry about making mistakes. If your mind starts to wander, gently bring it back to the coloring. Notice the details of the image and the colors you're using. When you've finished coloring the image, take a moment to appreciate your creation. Notice how you feel after completing the exercise.

The Color Conundrum

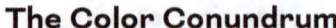

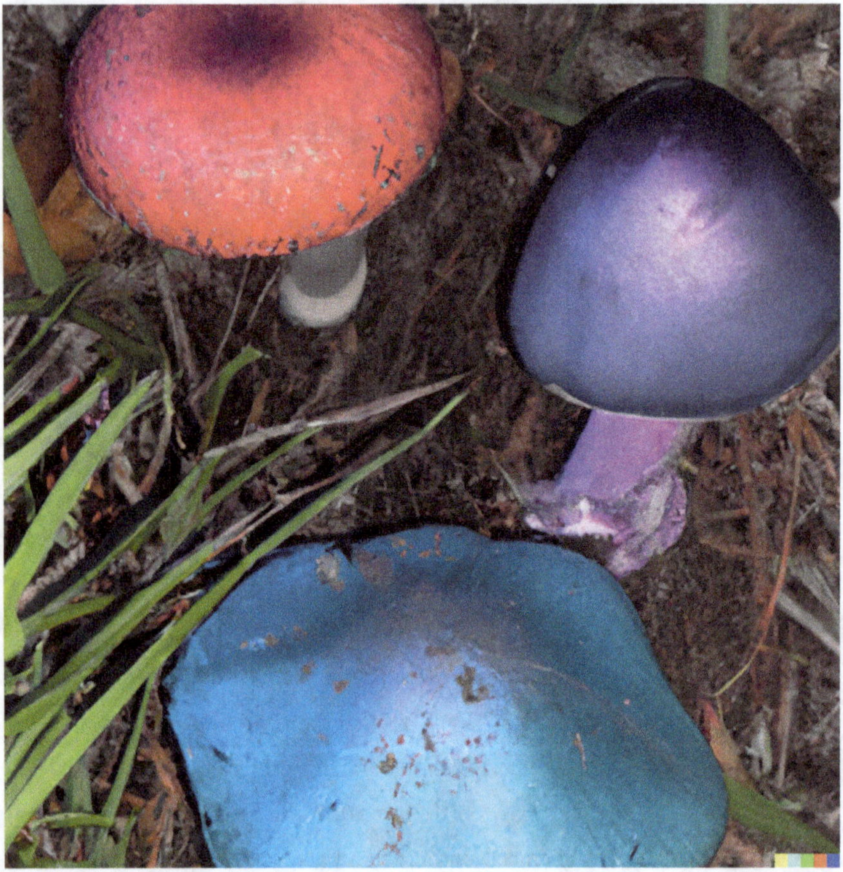

If blue mushrooms make you feel calm, and red mushrooms make you feel energized, what feelings might a purple mushroom evoke? How might this color combination symbolize the blending of different aspects of your life?

Self-expression Exercises

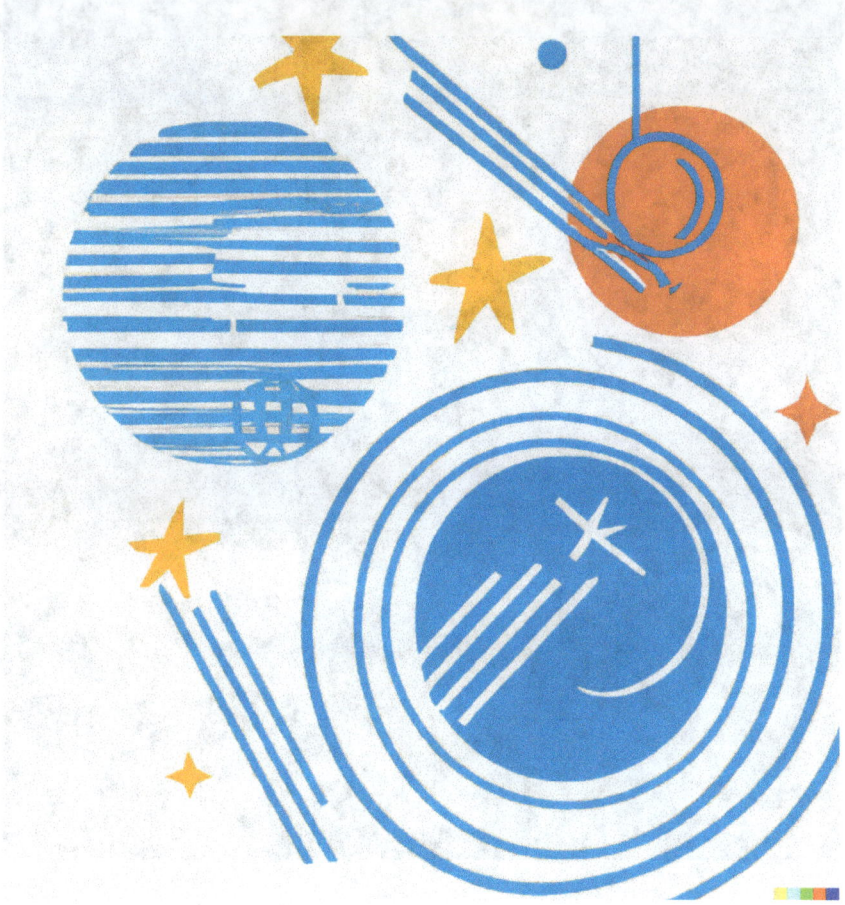

Create a visual representation of your journey using colors, shapes, and symbols. Consider how these elements might reflect your emotions, insights, or experiences.

159

Note to Self

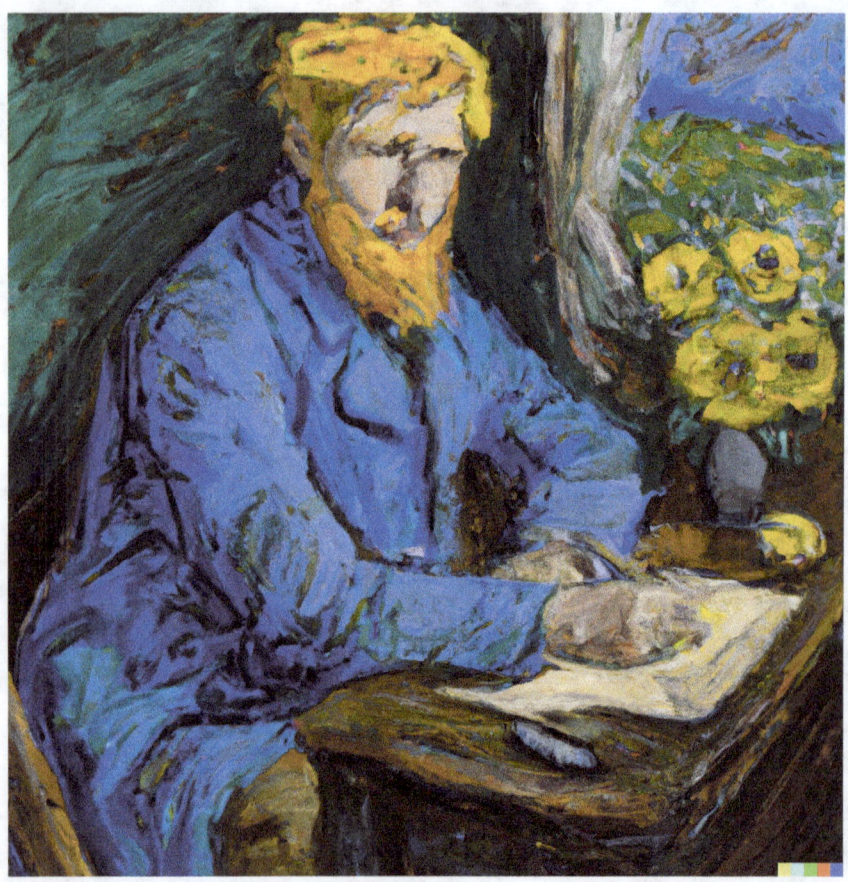

Describe the insights and lessons you've gained during your psychedelic experience. What advice or encouragement would you offer to your future self?

Mushroom Riddle

What has a cap but no head and can transport you to another world without moving an inch?

GLOSSARY

Afterglow: a residual positive feeling or sense of well-being experienced in the hours or days following a psychedelic journey.

Bad/Negative/Difficult/Challenging Trip: a negative or unpleasant experience during a psychedelic journey.

Closed-eye Visuals: visual hallucinations that occur when the eyes are closed.

Ego Death: a loss of sense of self or identity that can occur during a psychedelic journey.

Entourage effect: refers to the synergistic interaction of various compounds in a plant extract, such as cannabinoids and terpenes, that work together to produce a stronger overall effect than any one compound alone.

Entheogen: a substance that induces a spiritual or mystical experience.

Flashback: a re-experiencing of a previous psychedelic journey, often triggered by sensory stimuli or emotional states.

Hallucination: a perception of something that does not exist or is not present.

Integration: the process of incorporating insights and lessons from a psychedelic journey into daily life.

Magic Mushroom: a common term for mushrooms containing Psilocybin, a psychoactive compound.

Macrodosing: Refers to taking a larger, recreational dose of a psychedelic substance. Unlike microdosing, macrodosing involves taking an amount of a psychedelic substance that is sufficient to produce conscious-altering and profound effects on an individual's cognitive, emotional, and sensory experiences.

Microdosing: Refers to the practice of taking small, sub-perceptual amounts of a psychedelic substance, such as psilocybin, LSD, or mescaline, with the intention of experiencing subtle and beneficial cognitive, emotional, and sensory effects without the intensity of a full-blown "trip."

Mindset: the mental and emotional state a person brings to a psychedelic journey.

Mystical Experience: a feeling of interconnectedness or unity with the universe or a higher power.

Neurogenesis: the process by which new neurons, or nerve cells, are generated in the brain. This process is essential for learning, memory, and overall cognitive function.

Open-eye Visuals: visual hallucinations that occur when the eyes are open.

Mazatapec: a strain of magic mushrooms known for its visionary and euphoric effects.

Psilocybe Cubensis: a species of psychedelic mushroom that contains the psychoactive compounds psilocybin and psilocin. It is among the most widely distributed and popular species of magic mushrooms, known for its relatively easy cultivation and potent effects.

Psilocybe Cyanescens: a potent strain of magic mushrooms known for its intense and visual effects.

Psilocybe Mexicana: one of the oldest and most widely used strains of magic mushrooms, known for its euphoric and philosophical effects.

Psilocin: after the phosphorus chain decarboxylates from Psilocybin, it is converted into psilocin, which is the active compound that can cross the blood-brain barrier and produce psychedelic effects.

Psilocybin: the active alkaloid in magic mushrooms—a prodrug, which means it needs to be metabolized in the body to become active.

Psychedelic: a class of substances that have a profound and conscious-altering effect on perception, mood, thought, and sensory experiences. Examples of psychedelic substances include LSD, psilocybin (the primary psychoactive component in "magic mushrooms"), DMT, mescaline, and ayahuasca.

Set: the physical, mental, and emotional state a person brings to a psychedelic journey.

Setting: the physical, social, and emotional environment in which a psychedelic experience takes place.

Synesthesia: a perceptual phenomenon in which one sense is experienced in response to stimulation of a different sense.

Trip: in the context of psychedelic substances, a "trip" refers to the conscious-altering and often profound experience a person has after ingesting a sufficient amount of a psychedelic substance, such as LSD, psilocybin, or DMT.

Tripping: a common term for being under the influence of a psychedelic substance.

Unity Experience: a feeling of oneness or unity with the world or others.

Visionary Experience: a perception of vivid and meaningful images or scenes during a psychedelic journey.

NOTES